Cordel

THE SLIMMING SECRET

THE SLIMMING SECRET

by

Dr. S. KLINGER

PAPERFRONTS
ELLIOT RIGHT WAY BOOKS
KINGSWOOD, SURREY, U.K.

COPYRIGHT NOTICE

© Elliot Right Way Books MCMLXXII

© New edition. Elliot Right Way Books MCMLXXIV

Reprinted MCMLXXXII

All Rights Reserved. No part of this publication may be reproduced, stored in a retrieval system, or transmitted, in any form or by any means, electronic, mechanical, photocopying, recording or otherwise, without the prior permission of the Copyright owner.

SALE CONDITIONS

This book shall only be sold, lent or hired for profit, trade or otherwise in its original binding, except where special permission has been granted by the publishers.

While the author and publisher strive to ensure accuracy in this book, they regret they cannot be held responsible for any errors there may be.

Made and printed by Love and Malcomson Ltd., Brighton Road, Redhill, Surrey.

TO EDNA

ACKNOWLEDGMENT

Most of the calorie values are based on the figures given by R. A. McCance and E. M. Widdowson in The Medical Research Council Special Report Series No. 297 "The Composition of Foods" and are reproduced by kind permission of the Controller of H. M. Stationery Office.

CONTENTS

CHAPTER	PAGE
Foreword	9
Introduction	10
1. Is Fat Inherited?	12
2. Are Your Glands Responsible?	17
3. Do Fat People's Bodies Function Differently?	19
4. Does Fat Remain for Ever?	25
5. Are Salt and Water Fattening?	27
6. Errors in Slimming Tables	31
7. The Mystery of Hunger	36
8. Do Calories Count?	39
9. Sugar	54
10. "Slimming" Foods and "Slimming" Aids	62
11. Should We Believe the Advertisements?	77
12. Do Vitamins Help?	80
13. Do Drugs Help?	83
14. Unsound and Ineffective Slimming Methods	92
15. Difficulties in Slimming	115
16. The Slimming Secret	123
Index	158

Foreword

ON recovering from a serious illness due to obesity, I began at last to take slimming more seriously than I had done previously. While convalescing, I embarked on several years of study of weight-reducing and nutrition. Having met many contradictory, misleading and inaccurate assertions which could drive the would-be slimmer to give up in despair, I offer here a résumé of what I have learned from my studies and from my own experience as a doctor.

I have not dealt with all the erroneous ideas about the cause of obesity and methods of weight reducing, but I have covered many. Nor have I gone into great detail about nutrition. Leading works on this are always available in good libraries.

Some inaccuracies may have occurred in this book, for which I take full responsibility. I should be grateful for any helpful information from readers.

My special thanks go also to Professor McCance and Dr. Widdowson who permitted me to use the excellent calorie tables from their book "The Composition of Food", an adapted form of which is printed at the end with the permission of the Controller of H.M. Stationery Office.

I also wish to express my gratitude to my friend Mr. I. M. Hart for reading my manuscript and for his grammatical corrections.

Introduction

OBESITY has become a great problem in Western countries. According to recent observations, every fifth person in America and Britain is overweight. The situation in other developed countries is not much better.

Although the science of nutrition has made great progress during the last decades, the number of fallacies and wrong beliefs about the causes of obesity and the methods of slimming has also increased. Many fat people consider themselves victims of inheritance, of faulty glands or of improper function of their body. They have therefore lost the incentive to lose weight, after having made some attempts. Many have unsuccessfully used "miracle" cures which they have seen mentioned in books, magazines and newspapers. Some have fallen victims to advertisements which praised in glowing colours all sorts of miracle foods and gadgets which were supposed to melt away fat.

The slimming results of obesity clinics have also been very depressing. Patients, who started slimming with the earnest desire to lose their excess fat, gave up their attempts after a short time. Only a few were successful in reaching their normal weight, but a large percentage of these reverted to their original weight after a year or two. Only a few remained slim permanently.

Doctors listen daily to overweight patients, many of whom are obsessed with a conviction that they eat very little.

Fat people may brainwash themselves, but they cannot brainwash their own bodies. If they eat more than they need they will become fat, no matter how firmly convinced they are that they hardly eat anything. And they will not convince their bodies that some of the food they eat is free of calories. They may think that brown bread, margarine or diabetic jam and marmalade won't cause any gain in weight, that glucose can be safely added to tea or coffee, that cheese is a suitable food for slimmers, that lemon juice can melt away their fat, but the body will turn those "low calorie foods" into fat.

These misconceptions are the great enemies of fat people and prevent them from using the right road to a normal weight. No wonder that slimming results are so depressing.

Whether this book is going to improve these results remains to be seen. But if it can cure some fat people of their erroneous ideas; if it can show them more sensible ways of slimming, it will have served its purpose.

1
Is Fat Inherited?

"WHAT use is it for me to slim, if it is my nature to be fat?" is the frequent remark of overweight people. "If my parents and grandparents were fat, what chance have I to be different?"

So far no conclusive evidence proves that obesity is inherited, although some nutritionists still suspect a hereditary factor. One of the classic observations has been made by the American nutritionist Jean Mayer. He noticed that less than ten per cent of children living in Boston were fat when their parents were slim, but the incidence of obesity in children rose to 40% when one parent was fat and to 80% when both parents were. Some nutritionists considered this sort of observation as sufficient proof that there is a hereditary factor in overweight.

It is possible that heredity plays some part in obesity, but it cannot entirely be blamed for it. The nutritionist cannot watch the eating habits of children at home, but he can surmise. Is it not probable that fat children share the bad eating habits of fat parents? If parents eat high calorie foods, what choice has the child but to do the same? He has to eat what is on the table, although in the early years he is often rebellious and refuses to eat beyond his requirements.

I have often heard complaints from parents that their youngsters do not eat enough. But these children are usually well nourished and healthy. At an early age most

IS FAT INHERITED?

children have still the healthy instinct to eat only what they need. But in later years they succumb to the continuous urgings of the mother to eat beyond their requirements. Later, they begin to like high calorie foods which they rejected before. Even at the age of ten, children still have some healthy eating instincts which they gradually lose when they are forced to eat the wrong foods. For many years I have asked ten-year-old children whether they preferred fruit or puddings as the last course of a meal. Most preferred fruit. But most fifteen-year-old boys and girls favoured pudding. They had gradually acquired a taste for the higher calorie food which was given to them.

If one realises that a four ounce helping of suet pudding has a calorie value of 400, but an apple weighing four ounces has only 50, one can realise how much surplus food children consume in time. As well as pudding, cakes, biscuits and bread are frequently eaten in the homes of fat people. Children acquire a taste for them and finally like them just as much as their parents do.

Children of slim parents are not exposed to temptations to eat high calorie foods. Nor are they forced to eat pudding. They probably eat, like their parents, fruit or fruit salads as dessert.

Some nutritionists suspect a hereditary influence in obesity because of observation of various strains of animals in the laboratory. They noticed breeds of fat and thin mice and rats. But careful observation proved that fat animals either ate more food or were less active than the lean ones. Even the fat animals soon lost weight when their food intake was restricted or their activity increased. The installation of activity drums (big rotating cylinders), which the rats could enter or leave voluntarily, enabled the rats to multiply their movements. G. C. Kennedy, the American nutritionist, noticed that such rats ran as much as twenty to thirty kilometres a day. They were soon able to lose weight, which they could not do before because of their previously restricted activity.

Another line of research shows that generations of leanness did not prevent people from becoming fat, once their eating habits were altered. Very interesting observations were made in Israel, which, today, is a melting pot of Jews from all parts of the world. Among them are the Yemenite Jews who had been segregated from the "Western Jews" for approximately 2,000 years. When the Yemenites came to Israel more than twenty years ago, they were thin and wiry and differed much in their eating habits and activities from Jews who had come from Europe or America. Sugar, for instance, was a food which was hardly known among the Yemenites. In Israel they soon started to eat large quantities of sugar, although they still maintained some of their old eating habits. The consumption of sugar increased their body weight and caused a high incidence of diabetes and coronary thrombosis, diseases which were hardly known among them before.

There are several similar examples. In 1860, Indians were brought to Natal as labourers on the sugar plantations. They had lived in India under poor conditions and were not overweight. In Natal their situation improved and they were able to consume more sugar and fat than in their old home country. These new eating habits caused much overweight and many began to suffer from diabetes which had hardly been known previously.

Negroes in the United States of America, who are racially so close to the negroes in Africa, are heavier than their African brothers. The high calorie foods in America and the decreased activity there caused increased weight. Even in Africa, differences in weight have now been noticed between negroes living in rural regions and those living in towns. Negroes who settled in African towns got more opportunity to eat higher calorie food, especially sugar,

IS FAT INHERITED?

than those living in rural districts and soon began to gain weight.

Decreased activity can also play an important role. Observations have been made on the weight of the Irish living in the United States of America and of those in Ireland. Although the calorie intake of the Irish in their home country was higher, those in America were fatter. The native Irish worked mainly on farms, walked a lot or used bicycles to go to and from work. The American-Irish worked mainly in factories and used cars or buses for transport.

Similar observations were made on people living in the mountains or in valleys or towns. People living in the mountains of Switzerland or of South America were very active because they had to climb and carry heavy loads on steep mountain paths. Although they ate a lot, they were still found to be thinner than the town people, whose food intake was much smaller.

But even in towns body weight differs between physically active people and non-active people. It was found in London that bus conductors were lighter and less prone to coronary thrombosis than bus drivers. The bus drivers did not have the same opportunity as the conductors to move around or to walk up and down the stairs. Their body weight went up.

An interesting observation was made among women of various socio-economic status in New York. It was found that there were seven times more fat women in the lower classes than there were in the highest. Why? Did the poorer women inherit a greater tendency to obesity than the wealthier ones? Or did their glands function differently? No. They became fatter because they ate the same meals as their husbands. Men of the working class require a high calorie diet because of their physical activity. If their wives eat the same amount of food as their husbands, they are bound to gain weight because their physical activity is rarely as high.

On the other hand, upper-class men are physically less active than the working class, and require less food.

Let us finally look at one other example. During the last two wars, some European countries became short of food. Not only did the inhabitants of those countries become thinner, but the incidence of diabetes also dropped considerably. Fat people, who were forced to stay in prisoner-of-war or concentration camps, soon lost their excessive weight, *no matter how fat their ancestors had been.* No fat people left such camps at the end of the war.

It is therefore most unlikely that obesity is inherited. Environmental factors are almost certainly the main cause. If you want to get rid of your "traditional" obesity and become the ancestor of a new slim line, alter some of your "inherited" eating habits. Teach your children to eat the right food.

2
Are Your Glands Responsible?

A FAVOURITE excuse which many people find for their overweight is "abnormal function of their glands". It is often difficult for the doctor to rid the patient of that belief.

If asked *which* of their glands are deficient, such people have no idea. (In a very small minority of people the endocrine glands do cause overweight if they don't function properly. But in the vast majority of fat people the endocrine glands are functioning perfectly.)

Thus, people who suffer from overweight due to defective glands are rarities. If you are one of them, the medical profession would consider you a "highly interesting case".

Doctors, early in their career, are often inclined to refer patients of excessive weight (especially children) to specialists with the provisional diagnosis of glandular disturbance. Investigations usually prove that their glands function normally. Those children are fat because of their great intake of high calorie food, although their mothers rarely admit this.

At one time underfunction of the Thyroid gland was believed to increase the amount of fat in the body. Later investigations proved that the increase in body weight of people who suffered from that disorder was due to increase in water and not in fat.

Other glands which had once been considered to have some connection with the fat metabolism were the sex glands. The belief originated from the observation that castrated animals often increased in weight. Gain of body weight has also been noticed in human beings at particular stages of life, like puberty, pregnancy and menopause, when the functions of the sex glands changed. But castrated animals did not gain weight as long as they remained active. Stallions and bulls, which after castration were used for farm work, did not become fat.

Similar observations were made in human beings. Activity and intake of normal quantities of food prevented the incidence of obesity after the destruction of the sex glands. Some years ago, attempts were made to treat obesity with sex hormones but the results were negative.

Glands which do play an important part in the increase of weight are those which produce insulin. These are a group of small glands embedded in the pancreas, named Langerhans Islets after their discoverer. Occasionally these glands increase in size and produce more insulin than necessary. In such a state one experiences great hunger pangs which can only be relieved by taking larger amounts of carbohydrate.

Two other glands which may play a part in the cause of obesity are the pituitary glands and the suprarenal glands. The pituitary gland is a small gland at the base of the brain; the suprarenal glands are two glands which rest on the top of the kidneys. Excessive secretion of those glands *can* lead to obesity. But this is *extremely rare*.

All these glands have other functions apart from those referred to above, but it is beyond the scope of this book to go into further detail.

One person in five in the United States of America and Great Britain is overweight. If all those people suffered from improper functioning of their glands, the specialist would not consider the condition rare. It would be as common as a cold. So if you want to lose weight, forget your glands and start to eat properly.

3

Do Fat People's Bodies Function Differently?

WE often hear fat people say: "Look at Mr. and Mrs. So and So; they eat enormous quantities of food without ever getting fat. I eat like a bird* and I can't lose an ounce."

They think some people can utilise food better than others and that their bodies can burn excessive food without turning it into fat. But thorough research proves that a high intake of food without increased activity invariably makes you fat. It is just an easy excuse! If fat people were compelled to watch continuously the eating habits and activities of slim people, they would soon change their minds.

Thin people should not be judged by their intake of single meals eaten outside their homes. Don't go by what they are seen to eat in public.

The occupations of slim people should also be con-

---

*Incidentally, people who state that they eat like birds already commit an error of logic. If they could eat like birds, their gain in weight would be tremendous. A bird eats enormous quantities of food in proportion to its own weight. In a single day a bird may eat as much as half of its body weight. The bird's energy expenditure is very great and it has to eat great quantities of food to maintain its body. Most of the time it has to fly in order to move from place to place. This requires a lot of energy and, of course, a lot of food. The body temperature of a bird is also higher than that of a human being and requires great quantities of food for its maintenance. In order to utilise food quickly, the digestion of birds is much quicker than that of human beings.

sidered. If people do work which requires great physical activity, they need more food than do clerks. But even people of the same occupation may have different calorie requirements. Two clerks sitting at the same table may have different nutritional needs. Their activities outside their jobs may vary. One may go to work by car, the other may cycle or walk. One may read or watch television, the other may prefer gardening, cycling, playing golf, cricket or football, or may go swimming or dancing.

Age also plays an important part in the calorie requirements. A seventeen-year-old requires more food than a thirty-year-old, even if their activities are the same. In adolescence the body is growing fast and requires more food than at any other period of life.

One's size also plays an important part in one's food requirements. Tall people need more food than short if their activities are identical.

Climatic differences should also be considered. To keep the body temperature normal, more food is needed in arctic than in tropical regions.

Fever also increases the energy expenditure of the body. If the body temperature is raised, more body fat is burned, and a loss of weight takes place. The appetite is diminished or lost completely. It is therefore not surprising that people lose weight whilst ill.

There are stages in a woman's life when she requires more food than in normal times. During a pregnancy her calorie requirements rise steeply, because she has to feed both herself and the growing foetus. Even after the confinement the mother's calorie requirements may be greater than normal if she is breast-feeding her baby.

A person's weight influences his energy expenditure and consequently his calorie requirement. Two people of the same height, sex and age vary in their energy expenditure, if they do not weigh alike.

DO FAT PEOPLE'S BODIES FUNCTION DIFFERENTLY? 21

If two people of the same weight walk along the road, but one is carrying a case weighing 20 lbs. and the other nothing, it is obvious that the one carrying the case will use more energy and lose more weight than the other. If you are 20 lbs. overweight and you walk along with someone of normal weight (and the same height as yourself) your energy expenditure will also be greater than his because you carry with you 20 lbs. of superfluous fat. (The analogy between carrying a 20 lbs. case and 20 lbs. overweight is not strictly correct, because the fat in a human is distributed throughout the body and is easier to carry. An overweight of 20 lbs. therefore requires less energy expenditure than the carrying of a 20 lbs. case.)

This does not alter the fact that a heavy person expends more energy than one of normal weight, not only during walks but also when resting or even sleeping. The organs of fat people have to work harder than those of slim people. The heart has to pump the blood not only into the normal parts of the body but also into the superfluous fat. The lungs have to supply the additional fat with oxygen. The kidneys have to remove the excess fluid and the waste products not only from various organs of the body, but also from the additional fat. The stomach and the bowels also have no easy task with fat people. Such people usually eat bigger quantities of food which, to be digested, require more energy.

It is surprising that energy expenditure is so rarely considered when calculations are made on the gain or loss of body weight. A common fallacy observed by the American nutritionist Ancel Keys is the statement that the consumption of an additional slice of bread per day may cause a gain of 10 lbs. in body weight per year. According to this assertion, one should gain 100 lbs. in ten years. Of course, this does not happen. The body is not such a simple adding machine as some people try to make us believe. They forget that an increase in body weight causes an increase in energy expenditure which tends to counteract the gain in weight. If a person reaches a high body weight, he may eat great quantities of high calorie foods without gaining any more.

Equally wrong is the assurance, that a cut of 500 calories per day would cause a loss of 1 lb. body weight per week and 52 lbs. per year. The human body is not a simple subtraction machine either. If people lose weight, their energy expenditure decreases too, and the rate of weight loss is reduced.

Weight loss also depends on how overweight you are. A person who is 30 lbs. overweight would lose more weight per week on a cut of 500 calories than a person with an overweight of 5 lbs., because his energy expenditure is greater. Thus, the loss of weight diminishes once a heavy person becomes slimmer, in spite of his following the same diet as before.

The claims sometimes made that a certain 'miracle diet' is going to achieve a loss of so many pounds per week are just nonsense. The loss varies from person to person. If the weight of a person sinks below normal, the body takes measures to prevent further loss of weight. Energy expenditure decreases. At first, the person becomes weak and fatigues easily. Then he reduces his physical activity and is no longer able to run or to walk up steps quickly. Several internal changes take place too. The pulse rate falls and the blood pressure decreases. The body temperature also falls slightly and the activity of most organs diminishes. Such signs and symptoms were often seen in times of famine. But as long as the food supply was not too low, people still managed to live, although their working capacity was considerably restricted.

Another common misconception is spread by those who assert that a walk of a certain distance would cause the

DO FAT PEOPLE'S BODIES FUNCTION DIFFERENTLY?

loss of a certain amount of overweight. For example, we may be told that a walk of 30 miles would be necessary to lose 1 lb. in weight. Rather than walk 30 miles at once, it may be suggested that one should walk one mile daily, which would amount to 30 miles a month and a loss of 1 lb. during that time. Within a year the loss of 12 lbs. would be accomplished.

There are so many errors in these assertions that it is worth while discussing some of them. It is certainly not true that everyone would lose the same amount of weight in walking the same distance. Two people of different weights would lose different amounts of weight when walking a mile. The heavier person would lose much more than the lighter one. Curiously enough, even two people of the same weight and height may lose different amounts of weight by walking the same distance. A trained athlete who has been used to walking long distances will expend less energy and lose less weight than a beginner, who has not yet acquired the proper skill to walk long distances.

Another factor is the speed of the walk. It is obvious that more energy is expended on a quick walk than on a slow one; more weight is lost by walking fast. The level or the surface of the road is rarely considered; a walk on a hilly or rough road is certainly more tiring and more calorie-consuming than on the level. The weather or defects of the legs are other factors rarely mentioned.

This should not give the reader the impression that a cut of 500 calories per day or a walk of one mile is of little use to the slimmer. It is of great use. But it is worth knowing that the loss of weight does not occur according to some arithmetical formula. Neither does a cut of a certain amount of calories or a walk of so many miles per day cause the same loss of weight in every peron. Slimmers should therefore not be discouraged, if they notice during their course of slimming that they are losing less weight later than they did in the beginning, in spite of keeping to the same diet or to the same form of exercise.

There is one final misconception to be discussed. It is the assertion that a walk of half an hour is necessary to work off the weight gained by the intake of one slice of bread. We are also told about the many miles which we have to walk in order to burn the fat gained by a simple meal. That is, of course, not true. A person with an overweight of 40 lbs. will hardly gain any weight by eating a slice of bread because of his great energy expenditure. But he would lose weight by taking a brisk walk of half an hour. (However, as we shall see in Chapter 14, strenuous exercise is not advisable for a heavy person because of the strain it would impose on the heart.) Should a heavy person eventually become lighter he will need more exercise to lose the same amount of fat as before, because his energy expenditure has gone down with the decrease in his weight. Once he has reached his normal weight he will no longer lose any weight by walking his previous distances. But it is still necessary for him to continue his exercise and to live within his calorie limits in order not to gain weight again.

4

Does Fat Remain for Ever?

It is an old but erroneous belief that the fat tissue is an inactive and sluggish substance which cannot be disposed of once it has been acquired. Years ago nutritionists also thought that it was stagnant and dormant and could not be mobilised except by dietary deprivation. This accounts for the expression that "fat remains a lifetime on the hips".

The truth, however, is the reverse. Fat is a very active and lively substance which is quickly built up and mobilised in the body. There is a continuous turnover of fat tissue. People become fatter, not because new fat is added to the old, but because the newly built fat exceeds in quantity the old mobilised fat. People whose food intake is below calorie requirements become thinner, because the amount of newly built fat is less than the fat which has been lost.

These truths were discovered after 1946 when it became possible to study the chemical and physical changes in the body with the help of radioactive isotopes. Just as the discovery of X-Rays made it possible to look into the body and to observe the normal and abnormal appearances of various organs, so did the use of radioactive isotopes enable nutritionists to study normal and abnormal metabolism in the body. It is now possible to measure exactly the time taken to build the fat up and the time for its breakdown and disappearance. It has also been shown that the duration of fat varies in different parts of the body. Fat under the skin (depot fat), in the liver and intestines is much more quickly mobilised than the fat in the brain, which is chemically different.

Incidentally, radioactive isotopes enable us to study not only the metabolism of fat, but of other tissues too. It has been found, for instance, that a metabolism is going on in bone, and its speed can be precisely measured. Human bone tissue is replaced completely by new bone in about 200 days. There is a continuous coming and going in other tissues too. Fat has a very quick turnover, and in times of nutritional deprivation it is the first to be used up.

Perhaps, one day, a weight-reducing drug will be found with the help of radio-isotopes. As it is now possible to study the fat metabolism more precisely, it should become easier in future to investigate the effect of drugs upon it. So far, however, no safe drug has been found to speed up the fat metabolism. We still have to rely on dietetic measures to reduce our overweight.

5
Are Salt and Water Fattening?

SLIMMING is no easy task. It requires people to break off old eating habits, and to omit foods which they have enjoyed since childhood. Also one is daily exposed to all sorts of temptations. To watch other people in restaurants or at home eating appetizing, high calorie foods without being able to do likewise is a tantalizing experience.

This does not mean that the slimmer should burden himself with various unnecessary restrictions which are too often advised. One of these is cutting down on water and salt. It is an old and wrong belief that water and salt are fattening. In fact both compounds are free of calories. If you drink water and you go immediately afterwards on the scale your weight will be greater than before. If you take highly salted foods, and you then drink water to quench your thirst, your weight will also rise. But this increase in weight lasts only for a very short time, perhaps only for hours. Healthy kidneys soon excrete the superfluous water and salt.

The human body is very sensitive about water and salt. It does not tolerate any excess of either of them. Nor will it adapt itself to a loss of water and salt. In spite of the body's high water content (65%!) even a loss of 5% of water can cause various disturbing symptoms, such as burning thirst and inability to carry out work efficiently. Deprivation of 10% of body water causes severe illness, and a loss of 20%–25% water leads to death.

There is a great turnover of water and salt in our body. We lose water and salt continuously. Water leaves the body through the kidneys, bowels, lungs and skin. If we are exposed to great heat, we perspire heavily and we lose a large amount of water and salt through the skin. Miners, stokers, steelworkers, attendants in Turkish baths, etc., lose large amounts of water and salt during their working hours. If water and salt are not restored quickly, these workers may soon face muscle cramp. The cramp disappears soon after taking water and salt. Experienced miners have learned not to deprive their bodies of these two compounds for very long. They often drink fluids in the form of salted beer or salted barley water. Let this be a warning to those slimmers who are trying to cut down on water and salt when they have to perform heavy manual work in a hot atmosphere.

But even under normal conditions, it would be senseless to deprive oneself of water and salt. As we have learned above, a healthy body quickly expels superfluous water and salt. There is, therefore, no need for a slimmer, who has to give up so many of his treasured eating habits, to be condemned also to cut down on water and salt, and to eat insipid and unappetizing foods. Such restrictions are not going to encourage the slimmer to carry out the new diet for very long.

Slimmers should, therefore, be permitted to drink as much water as they desire. Water is not going to harm them. Unfortunately, some doctors still hold the opinion that slimmers should cut down the intake of water.

Fads and quacks have special rituals about drinking water. Some advise you not to drink water with meals, because water is supposed to dilute the gastric juice

ARE SALT AND WATER FATTENING?

and prevent the proper digestion of food. This is a fallacy because water actually stimulates the flow of gastric juice. Some will advise you to drink as little as possible.

It is fortunate that many slimmers, who think that they consume only a small amount of water, actually take more than they realize and so do not deprive themselves of the necessary amount. Water is not only consumed in the obvious form of drinks. It also enters the body with all sorts of foods.

Green vegetables and fruit contain about 90% water; root vegetables consist of 80% and meat of 50–70% water (lean meat has more water than fat meat). Even plain bread, which we usually call "dry" bread, is not as dry as we think. It may contain as much as 50% water. Apart from bread, pure carbohydrates, proteins and fats also contribute to the intake of water. They are oxidized in the body and yield a considerable percentage.

Just as it is wrong to deprive the slimmer of the intake of water, so it is equally wrong to drain away part of his body water artificially. Unfortunately, this is sometimes practised in order to reduce weight. It is either done by increasing perspiration (Turkish baths, etc.) or by stimulating the kidneys with the help of diuretic drugs. Perspiration and diuretics diminish only the water content of the body, but *not the fat*. Fat has only about 20% water, compared with other tissues such as those of the kidneys, muscles, skin, etc., which contain between 70–80% moisture. Even bone has about twice as much water as fat. Whichever tissue is going to lose water temporarily, fat tissue is certainly not going to be the one affected.

Diuretic drugs are of value only to water-logged patients, who, because of disease are not able to expel their superfluous water and salt. They are of no value to slimmers, who apart from their overweight, are in good health.

If you want to lose weight, try to lose not water, not salt, but fat. And do not deprive yourself of salt and plain water, try rather to avoid high calorie drinks such as beer, liqueurs, sweet mineral water, or tea and coffee sweetened with sugar.

6

Errors in Slimming Tables

IN any book or magazine article on slimming, take a look at the table which tells how much you should weigh at a particular height and at a certain age. Many of these tables make an allowance of additional weight for advancing age.

Although it is true that people do become heavier when they grow older, this still does not mean that an increase in weight in the course of years is normal or desirable, though the "middle-age spread" is unfortunately common. Modern textbooks on nutrition no longer make an allowance of extra weight after the age of twenty. Life insurance firms do not look favourably on clients who have steadily gained weight in later years, nor do their tables permit an increase in weight after twenty. But, unfortunately, we still find recently published works on slimming which reproduce tables granting an increase in weight.

Even the tables which allow no increase are still not quite correct. A person becomes fatter when he becomes older even if his weight has remained the same for many years. If a man of fifty weighs the same as he did when he was twenty, he has nevertheless become fatter. The reason for this is that some of his muscle tissue has been replaced by fat. In old age even part of his bone tissue becomes substituted by fat. People whose weight has remained stable for many years may notice that the size of their clothes has to be altered in the course of time. Men can no longer wear shirts of the same collar size, or trousers of the same waist line as they did in younger days although their weight has remained the same. Women at a later age find it impossible to wear the same size of clothes as before even if they have kept a steady weight during all those years.

To summarise, a person should weigh less than before in his later years, provided that his weight in his younger days was normal.

A mistake often made by people (and suggested by tables) is the belief that a "large frame" is an excuse for heavy weight. Many fat people console themselves that their overweight is due to heavy bones. It is true that a person with a large frame weighs more than a person with a small one, but the difference in weight is not as great as some people believe. Unfortunately, they are often aided in this mistaken belief by tables. Some of these give exaggerated allowances of extra pounds to people with "large frames". Here is an example taken from a table meant for a man six feet in height. It states that the man of a small frame should weigh between 148–158 lbs., of a medium frame between 154–170 lbs., and of a large frame between 168–181 lbs. When we look at both extremes, the difference in body weight of a man six feet high may be as much as 33 lbs. and still be considered normal. This, of course, is not correct. Bones are not as heavy as some authors suggest!

Let us look at a final misconception which is rarely considered. A person's weight may be above that stated in the tables, but he still need not be fat. An athlete

ERRORS IN SLIMMING TABLES

with a heavy bulk of muscles would normally weigh considerably more than a person with ordinary muscles. On the other hand, a person who does not use his muscles very much, may have part of his muscles replaced by fat, but, according to the tables he weighs less than he should. There are other conditions which may increase the weight of the body without showing signs of added fat tissue. Heart failure, disease of the kidney and liver can cause an accumulation of fluid in the body and considerably increase its weight.

Let us now consider tables which recommend certain daily dietary requirements for people of different ages and occupations; the figures are apt to be pretty much of a guess because it is impossible to work out a precise category for each individual.

These tables purport to tell us how many calories we need at a certain age and in a certain occupation. Some divide our types of work into light, medium and heavy, and recommend a higher intake of calories for the heavier type of work. But those estimates may not be accurate because it is often difficult to differentiate between various types of work. Other tables go into greater detail and give exact figures for the calorie requirements of various occupations. But even here it is impossible to give a precise figure. Take for instance, mining: a miner may be a face worker, mechanic or surface worker. Each differs greatly in energy expenditure. Does he work in a mine equipped with modern labour-saving devices or in a pit with old machines? It is obvious that the amount of work a miner has to perform varies greatly, but in tables he is just listed as a "miner" who requires so many calories per day.

Or let us look at the work of a farmer. Does he possess all sorts of modern machinery, or still use a plough and horses?

Little consideration is often given to the different energy expenditure of people working in the same industry. A person may be described as a textile worker, but his amount of work may be twice as much as that of his colleague who works in the same factory. One may be a supervisor who walks all the day in the factory checking the machines, another may stand all the time at the loom mainly using his hands and expending less energy.

Skill may also play an important part. An experienced factory worker uses less effort to do the same task than a beginner.

Finally, remember what was mentioned in Chapter 3. There are other factors which add to one's energy expenditure: different outside activities, age, weight of a person, etc., may also increase one's requirements for calories.

Interesting, but very debatable, are the figures which tell us of the amount of protein which we require daily. Several authorities on nutrition have agreed that an average 70 kg. (11½ st.) adult male requires 1 gram of protein daily per kilogram of bodyweight (1 oz. per 4½ st.), but it is questionable whether that is sufficient.

Protein is a very important foodstuff. It is a vital part of all living cells, and it is constantly required for the repair and growth of the body tissues. The body cannot store large amounts of protein, but without a sufficient supply would soon break down.

It is generally assumed that increased muscle activity does not cause a breakdown of body protein, and, therefore, that an additional supply of protein should not be necessary. The extra energy used during greater physical activity would be covered by the calories of fats and carbohydrates. But this assumption is doubtful.

A car, for instance, which is used more, not only needs more fuel but is also bound to undergo greater wear and

ERRORS IN SLIMMING TABLES

tear. In the same way, a human body which does harder work is likely to need more protein.

There are also other circumstances which demand more protein, such as burns, fractures, damage of the liver, some diseases of the kidneys, pregnancy and lactation. Growing children and adolescents also demand a lot of extra protein.

There is an interesting controversy about the quantity of protein needed in a hot climate. E. G. Holmes, an Australian nutritionist, points out the increased loss of Nitrogen through perspiration in hot weather and advises people to eat more protein under such circumstances. But other experts are of the opinion that the increased consumption of protein in a hot climate increases the production of heat in the body, due to the "specific dynamic action" of protein, and they find it advisable to eat less protein under such conditions.

Another argument is the amount of protein needed in old age. One view is that the call for protein in old age is less than at any other time of life. Other specialists take the view that the bodies of old people undergo a greater wasting of the tissues, and they recommend a higher intake of protein.

The foregoing may lead the reader to wonder what value there is in the tables published in books and articles on nutrition or slimming. Some of the tables are of great importance, especially those dealing with the composition and the calorie values of food. These are the slimmer's best guide out of the abyss of obesity.

7
The Mystery of Hunger

"How can I resist the temptation to eat when I am always so hungry?", is a frequent question. But are you really hungry as often as you think? When are you actually hungry? Your answer will probably be: "As soon as my stomach is empty". Often this is so. But does an empty stomach necessarily cause hunger?

When you wake up in the morning your stomach is empty, but do you have that gnawing hunger? Many people work before breakfast, and do not feel hungry. At other times, absorbed in work or reading an interesting book, one may completely forget that a meal is ready.

In some emotional states there is no desire to eat even if the stomach has been empty for several hours. Fear, worry and severe depression can take away the appetite.

Similar observations have been made in animals. Even after a long spell of fasting, some animals do not eat if they are disturbed by strangers. A dog which has been without food for twenty-four hours and will then eat greedily, often stops eating if he is watched by an unfamiliar person. Farmers have often seen that cows in sheds stop eating in the presence of strangers.

Consider the desire for food in times of illness. If you are in bed with a high temperature, you rarely feel hungry.

THE MYSTERY OF HUNGER

Here is a fact which has long puzzled physiologists and nutritionists. *People who are without food for some time gradually lose the sensation of hunger.* Provided they have enough water, some people manage to live for weeks without food. Contrary to what you would expect, those who have survived long periods of abstinence declare that the sensation of hunger disappeared after the first two or three days. This is an interesting phenomenon for which no physiological explanation has so far been found.

This is why some prisoners have been able to carry out hunger-strikes for a considerable time. After the first two or three days of discomfort, they probably did not feel their subsequent ordeal to the extent one would have expected.

These observations encouraged some nutritionists to carry out fasting cures for people with gross overweight. Some patients managed to lose considerable weight during long periods of fasting. More about this in Chapter 14 (page 92).

An empty stomach, therefore, does not necessarily make you feel hungry. But what about a full stomach? Normally, this should give you a feeling of satiety, but does it always do so? Some people, at certain times of day, feel hungry even if the stomach is fairly full. If you are accustomed to having tea or coffee, perhaps with a few biscuits, at mid-morning, you will feel hungry if you cannot have your snack, even though you have had a good breakfast. Physiologists make a distinction between hunger and appetite. They define appetite as a desire for some special food, and hunger as the craving to eat anything. Physiologists do not, therefore, consider a person to be hungry if his stomach is full, but it is not easy to draw the line.

The feeling of hunger can be conditioned by time,

whether the stomach be empty or full. If you expect a meal at a certain time, you will feel hungry shortly before it. Many people would be very hungry if they had to miss their midday meal, even if they had had a substantial breakfast. But the same people would not be so hungry if they had made up their minds to fast for a day.

Similar observations on time-conditioned hunger have been made in animals. Have you ever watched a lion in a zoo before feeding time? He becomes restless, paces up and down in his cage and settles down again only when given his meat. During his years of captivity he has learned from experience that food is served at regular intervals, and he becomes restless and hungry when feeding times arrive. Then his stomach is probably empty, but would that lion feel just as hungry at regular intervals if he were in his natural environment? There he would sometimes have to go for days without food. The restlessness is really nothing more than a response to a time stimulus.

The cause of hunger and its control are still not fully understood. Perhaps the future will reveal more of this mystery. It will then be easier to find better methods of slimming than those practised today.

8
Do Calories Count?

WHAT is a Calorie?

It is a unit of energy or heat. In scientific terms it is the amount of heat required to raise the temperature of 1,000 grams of water by 1 degree Centigrade. To do this we would usually use fuels such as wood, coal, paraffin, petrol, gas, electricity, etc. But we could also heat water by burning food, such as bread, butter, cheese, etc. It is obvious that a certain quantity of margarine, butter or oil will produce more heat when burned than will the same weight of bread. On the other hand, the amount of heat obtained by burning a certain weight of bread will exceed that obtained from the same weight of cabbage, cauliflower or any other green vegetable.

Any food gives off a certain amount of heat when burned. To find out the exact amount of heat which various foods deliver, scientists use a special vessel called a *bomb calorimeter* in which the food is burned and the amount of heat measured. The more heat food gives off, the higher is its calorie content.

Just as engines need fuel to keep them going, so does the body need fuel for its organs to function. The fuel of the body is food. Food is necessary to keep the body at a steady temperature (98.4° F.), to supply the body with energy and to provide its tissues with substances for their upkeep and growth.

If food is taken in excess, or, as nutritionists term it,

in greater calorie quantities than required, the superfluous calories are stored in the body in the form of fat. In short, calories taken in excess cause obesity. Many people do not know the calorie value of foods and have little idea of what to cut down. They have gained weight throughout the years without having been aware of the high number of calories they have been consuming. No wonder that fat people often think that they eat very little.

Ignorance of the calorie content of food can sometimes have disastrous effects. I remember a bus driver who once asked me for advice about his sudden increase in weight. He had gained over twenty pounds within a year, and was now finding it difficult to sit in the driving seat of his bus. The increase in weight had started about a year earlier, soon after the death of his wife. He was convinced that the shock of his bereavement had disturbed his glands which were responsible for his sudden increase in weight. A careful inquiry about his present eating habits did not at first reveal anything. He remained adamant that he still ate the same as he had eaten before. He firmly denied that he had lately indulged in any additional intake of food. When finally I asked him whether he now drank more tea or coffee than before, he admitted that since the death of his wife he spent his lonely evenings drinking several cups of sweetened tea. After further inquiries I found out that he drank about fifteen cups of tea daily, and sweetened each with two teaspoonfuls of sugar. "But tea is no food," he said innocently. Little did he know that the thirty teaspoonfuls of sugar which he consumed with the tea contained approximately 900 calories. The milk in the tea had added another 300 calories to his intake. No wonder that he had gained weight so rapidly through adding 1,200 calories daily to his ordinary food. Had he sweetened his tea with saccharine, he would have saved 6,300 calories weekly, a considerable number.

How Harmless are Snacks?

Overweight people rarely disclose to doctors what they have taken between their meals. Do they really think that snacks have no calories? If only people knew more about the calorie content of some snacks, they would be more careful. Consider the following example: A woman, after a busy shopping trip, goes into a snack bar, just for a cup of tea. Unfortunately, snack bars offer more than tea or coffee. They display varieties of cakes and sandwiches. In a weak moment she takes a small piece of cake and decides to have coffee instead of tea. But she does not know that the small piece of cake weighing about two ounces may contain as many as 300 calories. The coffee is probably mostly milk flavoured with a dash of coffee (many snack bars serve coffee made this way), and so she adds another 120 calories to those in the cake. But this is not all. Sugar is the only item in snack bars which can be taken in any quantity at no extra cost. Each teaspoonful of sugar means another 30 calories. She finally leaves the snack bar after an intake of at least 450 calories. Does she ever tell the doctor about her visit to the snack bar? Hardly ever. Why? Because she has no idea that this small and "innocent" snack contained so many calories.

Some fat people have told me that they never eat cakes and are still overweight. But after questioning they have admitted that they eat bread with butter or margarine. At breakfast they often add to this, marmalade, an egg, sweetened tea or coffee.

What does a cake consist of? Mainly flour, eggs, sugar and fat. The same ingredients, really. The body does not discriminate between a cake and the combination of bread, fat, marmalade and an egg. It splits foods into the same final components, no matter how they were prepared, and turns them into fat if they have been taken in excessive quantities. Do not therefore imagine that if you eat bread with the usual additions, your calorie intake is different from that of a cake.

Unsuccessful Slimmers Who "Never Have Breakfast"

Although many fat people admit to having breakfast, there are many others who deny it. The majority of statements are not correct. Most fat people who have not had breakfast take high calorie snacks in the mid-morning. What they are really doing is to take a delayed breakfast. It is again the old story that foods taken outside mealtimes are not considered to be meals and are thought to be free of calories. In clinics I have often had long talks with people who "never had breakfast". Only after much insistent questioning did they reluctantly admit that they took snacks in the mid-morning. The calorie value of some of these snacks would have put a good breakfast to shame!

How Slim People Stay Slim

It is one thing to listen to the statements of obese people about their eating habits, but even more interesting to learn from lean people about their ways of eating. Just as fat people claim that they eat very little, so do thin ones tend to say that they eat like horses. But when they are asked how much pudding or how many cakes they eat daily, they usually admit that they do not touch either of them. Thin people, especially adults, very often detest sweet foods. Chocolate, cakes, sugar and other sweet foods are often repugnant to them. They never drink tea or coffee sweetened with sugar. Considering that the British consume over two pounds of sugar per head

DO CALORIES COUNT?

weekly one can see how many calories thin people omit by not taking sugar. But by avoiding sugar lean people are also saved from the intake of other high calorie foods. Sugar is rarely taken in its pure form. It is often combined with foods such as flour and fat, e.g. in cakes, puddings, biscuits, etc. These foods are well known for their high calorie content.

Apart from sweet foods, thin people do not eat great amounts of bread, either.

There is another interesting feature of lean people, especially women. They feel "full" after eating only small quantities of food. When I asked thin women about their eating habits, they usually told me that they ate well. But after a few more questions they disclosed that for breakfast e.g. they had hardly more than a slice of toast and a cup of unsweetened tea. Thin people also rarely eat between meals.

Here is another interesting fact which can be seen daily in snack bars: some slim women do not require more than a sandwich and a cup of tea or coffee for their midday meal. We have learned before that such a snack eaten between meals can add considerably to the daily calorie intake. But, eaten as a main meal without taking anything else in the mid-afternoon, that snack is not of such great calorie significance. I myself could not eat a meal which has so little bulk. I should be hungry before even leaving the door of the restaurant. But some people, apparently, are satisfied with such small meals. It is difficult to understand why. The mystery of the sensation of hunger has still not been solved.

Thin people are certainly to be envied. They do not need to know the calorie value of foods in order to remain slim. They either do not like high calorie foods or they eat some, such as bread in very small quantities.

I have seen lean labourers who could hardly read or

write, but they were shining examples of proper eating habits, without having the faintest idea of calories. I have also seen obese highly intelligent university graduates, who, in their eating habits, behaved like morons. Knowledge of the calorie value of foods could have liberated them from their overweight.

Some Pitfalls due to Ignorance of Calorie Values.

For fat people who want to lose weight, a sound knowledge of the calorie content of foods is essential. Fortified by this knowledge, they can soon shed their superfluous weight, and, what is even more important, retain a stable weight afterwards. We have already seen how many calories there are in some snacks eaten between meals. But what about the calories consumed at main meals?

Diners often have the notion that foods which do not taste sweet contain only a few calories. Fat patients often tell me that they eat only unsweetened puddings, or cakes with very little sugar. But these puddings and cakes still have a high calorie content because of the amount of flour and fat in them.

This is also true of other foods. They have heard that fish and meat can be safely eaten because proteins are less easily converted into fat than are carbohydrates. But how often is fish or meat so prepared that it can safely be eaten by the slimmer? Fish, grilled, boiled or steamed is a very good food for those who want to lose weight. Unfortunately, fish is rarely prepared this way. A four ounce helping of steamed haddock contains about 84 calories, but the same quantity of fried haddock has 184 calories. And do people eat fried fish as a single dish? Only rarely. A popular addition to fried fish in this country is "chips". These small pieces of fried potatoes add very many calories to the meal. Fish cakes are perhaps worse. They may contain up to 244 calories in four ounces.

People think that fish cakes consist almost entirely of fish, but they include other ingredients such as potatoes, eggs, bread crumbs, flour and fat, most of which have a high calorie value.

So it is with lean meat. When grilled or boiled, it is a suitable food for slimmers. But lean meat is expensive. The cheaper cuts often contain a considerable amount of fat and here there is a vast difference in calories. Fat meat may contain more than twice as many. When meat is cooked, it is not often easy to differentiate between the fat and the meat, because fat loses its distinctive colour when heated. If you want to see how much fat there is, for example, in pork or lamb, look into a butchers' shop window. You will see the distinctive white colour of fat contrasting sharply with the red meat and get some idea of how much fat you have eaten unawares in the past.

The Hidden Danger in Meat Foods

There are some dishes, described as meat dishes, which have little to do with meat. Steak puddings, Shepherd's pie, steak and kidney pies, especially when prepared with an eye to economy, often contain only small quantities of meat. They have more flour, fat or potatoes than meat.

Another problem is sausages. Here again some may think that by eating beef or pork sausages, they mainly eat beef or pork. It is well known that sausages contain some bread, but few realize that sausages also contain a large proportion of fat. You can see part of the fat in a sausage by trying a little experiment which a hospital dietician once showed me. Take a beef or pork sausage, punch some holes into it with a fork, and put the sausage on a metal plate under a hot grill. Remove the grilled sausage after a few minutes, and tilt the plate, so that the hot liquid fat that comes out of the sausage can run down into the lower part of the plate. Keep the plate in this position until the fat becomes cold and more visible. You will be surprised to see how much has come out. But this is not all the fat of the sausage. There is still some fat left in it. Most people, however, do not grill sausages, but fry them. By this method, they not only leave all the fat in the sausage, but even put in extra.

Can One Slim on a High Fat Diet?

Some authorities maintain that a high fat diet does not cause obesity. Only carbohydrates are supposed to be the cause of overweight. Here we touch on a controversy which arose in 1956 after an observation made by two nutritionists Kekwick and Pawan. They found that obese patients, treated for several weeks in hospital, lost more weight on a fat diet than on a carbohydrate diet, although the fat diet contained more calories than the carbohydrate diet. Soon after the publication of this, newspaper and magazine articles began to advocate a high fat diet for the reduction of weight. Some also claimed that the intake of fat did not cause obesity.

Many nutritionists opposed all these assertions by pointing out that over a long period the reduction in a person's intake of fat or of carbohydrates resulted in the same loss of weight as long as the number of calories was cut down. That so many people initially lost more weight on a fat—than on a carbohydrate diet was due, in the opinion of some nutritionists, to the difference in the water balance. They believed that a fat diet, taken for a short time, released more water from the body than a carbohydrate diet.

Whatever may be the outcome of this controversy, it would still be safer for the slimmer to cut down not only on carbohydrates, but also on fats. We must not forget that in countries where obesity is very common, fat is eaten in great quantities. For example, in the U.S.A., where every fifth person is overweight, 40% of the calorie intake is fat.

Misconceptions about the Calorie Value of Certain Foods

Eggs

Eggs, because of their great nutritional value, are often thought to be high calorie foods; other foods are often underrated. Ask people how many medium sized biscuits (crackers) are equivalent to one egg. You will usually hear the most surprising estimates. I have often been told 'at least half a dozen'. My informants have then always been surprised to learn that a single medium sized biscuit contains about the same number of calories as an egg.

Potatoes

A food whose calorie value is greatly overestimated. John McKenzie, who has done a lot of research into the eating habits of people in Great Britain, found that the vast majority regarded the potato as the most fattening food of all. 62% of housewives thought that potatoes should be avoided when slimming, but only 5% of them believed that biscuits should be omitted in order to lose weight. Yet, weight for weight, biscuits contain at least six times as many calories as potatoes! In fact, of 15 different foods which have far more calories than potatoes housewives still considered potatoes to be the most fattening.

Potatoes are not as fattening as many believe, as long as they are eaten the right way. A four ounce potato contains only 80 calories. About 30 calories more than an apple of the same weight. If you eat a sensible meal, such as lean meat or fish with two or three low calorie vegetables, and you add to these a medium sized potato, you are, from a dietary standpoint, not committing such a great sin as some people may try to tell you.

Why is the calorie value of a potato not high? Because it is 80% water which has no calorie value. The rest of the potato consists of starch, minerals, a small amount of protein and some of the vitamins B and C.

Why, then, do so many slimming diets ban potatoes? Because most people do not prepare potatoes suitably for the slimmer. Potatoes boiled, baked in their jackets, or steamed, are no menace to the slimmer because of their low calorie content. But do many of us eat potatoes so prepared? Unfortunately not! Chips, for example, contain three times as many calories as plain potatoes. But this is not the end of the story. Very few people eat only 4 ounces of chips at a meal. 8 ounces or even more are often eaten at a time. This means it is not unusual to consume at least 500 additional calories when taking chips with a meal. Can you see now why doctors usually forbid potatoes to slimmers, who are so rarely familiar with calorie tables?

Another potato dish often eaten at home and in restaurants is creamed potatoes. Here the calorie value depends on the amount of fat or milk which is added to the potatoes.

Let us finally look at a seemingly harmless potato preparation which is often eaten absentmindedly when watching television; potato crisps. Remember that owing to the frying oil, a packet of potato crisps weighing only 2 ounces contain more than 300 calories. Quite a significant number for a tit-bit.

Soups

Do you realize now why it is so important to know the calorie value of foods? Not only potatoes, but numerous other foods may vary in their calorie value according to the way they are prepared. Consider soups. A plain chicken or meat soup contains only a few calories if the fat is skimmed off. But the calorie value of a thick soup, made with flour, fat and several other fattening ingredients, may rise steeply. If you eat bread with it, as is so commonly done, you add even more.

Cheese

Many people are under the impression that cheese is not fattening. Some have even been shown diet sheets for slimming, where cheese was not among the forbidden foods. It is often said that cheese does not contain carbohydrates and can therefore safely be eaten by slimmers. Some people even believe that cheese is a pure protein food which is always permitted to slimmers.

It is true that most cheeses contain only traces of carbohydrates and nearly 25% protein, but they also contain fat which nearly always exceeds the amount of protein. 4 ounces of Cheddar cheese contains about 480 calories. Other cheeses have not many calories fewer. Some, such as cream cheeses, Gruyere, or the Norwegian cheese Mysost, have even more. Cheese should only be eaten in very small quantities. A daily intake of 4 ounces of cheese would add 3,000 calories to your weekly consumption.

Price is no Measure of Calorie Value

It is dangerous fallacy for the slimmer to think that cheap foods have a low calorie value. Take meat. The fatter the meat, the cheaper it is, but the greater also is its calorie content. So it is with bacon. Fat bacon costs far less than lean, but it can sometimes contain twice as many calories. Herring is one of the cheapest of fish, but is highest in calories. Compare the prices of bread and lean beef. A pound of bread contains about 1,120 calories and a pound of lean steak 800 calories, but what a difference in price! There are, of course, exceptions. Some of the low calorie vegetables, such as asparagus, are very expensive. Fresh fruit, a suitable food for the slimmer, is not cheap either. But there are more cheap high calorie foods than dear ones.

A low calorie diet with some variety can therefore be rather expensive, especially when some of the fruits and vegetables are out of season. But, one can always look for ways of reducing the cost.

Are Awkward Calculations and Weighing of Foods Necessary?

It is not true that after learning the calorie values of foods, constant weighing and involved calculations of food portions is necessary. The reason for this is very simple. Once you become acquainted with the calorie values, you will find it unnecessary to weigh. Whether you have eaten $3\frac{1}{2}$ ounces of pudding or 4 ounces makes little difference to you. You have eaten a high amount of calories. On the other hand, it does not matter whether you add several ounces of low calorie vegetables to your meal. The few calories you add by eating additional low calorie vegetables are of no importance.

Once you have weighed a slice of bread you will be able to estimate the approximate quantity of calories in it. You will also learn to measure the amount of calories which are, for instance, in fruit, without using scales. A medium sized apple weighs about 4 ounces and has about 50 calories. It is of little consequence for the slimmer if he eats an apple which weighs an additional ounce. The intake of 10 or 15 more calories is unimportant.

It is often impossible to weigh foods and to calculate their correct calorie content. Meals eaten in restaurants

DO CALORIES COUNT? 51

cannot be weighed by the diners nor is it possible to know the amount of all their ingredients. But even here, knowledge of the calorie values will be of great help to you. You will choose the lesser evil and avoid eating high calorie foods such as chips, pies, puddings, etc.

I have not used my food scales for working out calorie values for many years.

Willpower and Slimming

It is often believed that knowledge of the calorie values of foods is of little use without strong willpower. I disagree. From my own experience I know that knowledge of the calorie contents of foods has helped me to resist eating high calorie foods without much exertion of willpower. How many of us know that a 4 ounce portion of pudding contains about 400 calories, whereas an apple of equal weight has only 50? Yes, pudding is eight times more fattening than apple. I have substituted an apple or other fresh fruit for puddings for years and have saved over 2,000 calories a week. You could do the same.

Individual Calorie Requirements Vary

People often want to know how many calories they have to eat daily in order to lose their overweight and then to remain permanently slim. It is impossible to name a figure because calorie requirements vary from individual to individual as shown in Chapter 3.

Scientists have used all sorts of methods to measure the energy expenditure and calorie requirements of various individuals. Many years ago "Respiration Chambers" were used in order to measure calorie output. People were put in special chambers in which all their energy expenditure was measured. In later years these chambers were replaced by a portable apparatus. One type was the

"Planck Respirometer" which weighed about 5 lbs. and had to be carried by a person in order to measure his calorie output. One of the latest instruments for measuring a person's energy expenditure is the size of a small cigarette box.

How to Keep Within Your Calorie Needs

These methods of measuring calorie output are time-consuming and expensive. In practice, it is not necessary for the slimmer to know *how many* calories he requires per day. It is of greater importance for him to know whether he has eaten within his calorie requirements. If he has gained weight after a time, it is obvious that he has eaten above his calorie requirement. If he has lost weight, he has eaten below his requirement. *It is as simple as that.* A scale will replace all these expensive pieces of apparatus. Weigh yourself every week and you will see whether you have eaten more or less than you need.

Is It Difficult To Learn Calorie Values?

A final question: "How do I become familiar with the calorie values?" There is no need for learning calorie values to be a tedious task of memorizing endless tables of dry figures. Here I can talk again from my experience. I hate figures. Memorizing is a nightmare. When I started slimming years ago and realised the importance of calories I wrote about 500 figures in a small notebook. During the first few weeks of slimming I consulted this book daily for a few minutes after each meal and snack. I was amazed to see the high calorie content of some of the foods I had eaten that day and in the past. Gradually I came to understand calorie figures without having to memorize them and learned to avoid high calorie foods.

Within a year I lost all my overweight, and my weight has remained stable for the last 11 years.

In brief: acquaint yourself with calorie values. Calories do count!

9
Sugar

THE consumption of sugar in Great Britain has gone up 25 times during the past two hundred years. In 1770, only 4 lbs. of sugar were eaten in a year per head of the population. This figure rose to 10 lbs. in 1830, to 60 lbs. in 1880, reached 100 lbs. at the beginning of this century and has now risen to over 120 lbs. Over 2 lbs. of sugar per week! In calories this means about 600 calories daily, or over 4,000 per week. A substantial figure! But ask a fat person how much sugar he eats in a week and he will either deny eating any or admit to only a small fraction of the statistical average. Where then does all the sugar go?

The paradox is solved by the fact that fat people only count the sugar which is visible to them taken out of the sugar bowl for sweetening tea or coffee or sprinkled over various foods. They seem to forget the sugar which is hidden in so many prepared and manufactured foods. About a third of the contents of plain cakes, for instance, is sugar. Rich cakes with fillings and icing are, of course, made with a far greater amount. Sweet pies, biscuits, jellies, jams, marmalades, candies and chocolates are loaded with it. Jams contain about 70% and chocolates usually 50% sugar.

Canned fruits vary in their content of sugar, depending on whether ordinary, heavy, or extra heavy syrup has been included in the tin.

Manufactured soft drinks, such as carbonated or concentrated fruit drinks, also contain plenty of sugar. So do manufactured savoury foods such as tomato and other sauces, mayonnaise, salad cream and pickles. Canned soups and vegetables, and even peanut butter are not free from sugar.

And there are many more sugar-containing manufactured foods.

The statistics tell us of an annual consumption of over 120 lbs. of sugar per head. But this applies only to cane or beet sugar (both are chemically identical). We also eat other types of sugar which are not included in these statistics. Honey, for instance, consists of fruit sugar and glucose. Although these are chemically different from table sugar, they are still utilized by the body in the same way, and contain a high number of calories.

Other sugar-containing foods, not included in the statistics, are fruits which are eaten in great amounts. Apples, pears, peaches, damsons, Victoria plums contain about 10% sugar, bananas 20%, dried apricots 40%, dried figs and peaches 50%, dried currants and sultanas 60%. All these sugars are chemically not identical with cane or beet sugar but the body uses them in the same way.

Sugars are not necessarily sweet tasting substances. Milk, for instance, contains a type of sugar (milk sugar or lactose) which has hardly any sweet taste. As most of us drink milk daily, the amount of milk sugar thus consumed is substantial. This form of sugar is also not included in the above statistics.

To take the matter further, the starches of all cereals or cereal-containing foods are also turned into sugar in the body. This sugar is then either converted into glycogen and stored in the liver and muscles or else used up for energy, or turned into fat. Starches consist of several groups of sugar and are broken down to simple sugars during the process of digestion. Whether you eat sugar or starch makes little difference to the body. Each is converted into simple sugars inside the body and these are then absorbed into the bloodstream, but the conversion of table sugar is much quicker.

In short, the amount of sugar per head of the population utilized by the body in a year is really far greater than 120 lbs.

Normally it is difficult to adapt oneself to new types of foods, but sugar seems to be an exceptional case. People who have not previously known sugar (or used it very sparingly), become quickly adapted to it if they settle in a country where sugar is freely available. A classical example is the Yemenite Jews who had hardly known sugar in their old country but quickly became used to it when they settled in Israel. After a relatively short time, owing to their large consumption of sugar, they began to suffer from degenerative diseases such as diabetes, coronary thrombosis, etc.

Similar observations have been made on Indians who had settled in South Africa to work on sugar plantations. Within a few years of arrival there, their sugar consumption had rapidly increased, and many of them also began to suffer from diseases such as diabetes, etc., which were hardly known among them when they lived in India.

Even Eskimos have found sugar very palatable, although traditionally they are mainly used to living on fat and protein. Fortunately for them, the amount of sugar they are eating at present is still very low, so that they are not yet in danger of suffering from diseases caused by a large intake of sugar.

It has always puzzled nutritionists why sugar has had

such a great appeal to people. Compared with the vast number of people who like sugar, there are only a few who dislike it. Curiously enough, there also exist people who detest some sweet foods, but like other foods made with plenty of sugar.

We all know people who dislike tea sweetened with sugar but who eat sweet cakes or biscuits with their tea. We know that porridge is eaten with sugar in England, but with salt in Scotland. Nevertheless, the Scots are just as fond of sugar as the English. Scottish fruit cakes, shortbreads, puddings, etc., contain plenty of it.

Sugar has not always been the cheap commodity that it is now. It was once a very rare and expensive food. Indeed it was not used as a food in the beginning but as a spice. Much later it was treated as a food by a few, very wealthy people. The nutritionist Passmore tells us that in the thirteenth and fourteenth centuries the price of a pound of sugar was more than the week's wages of a servant. Even in later centuries, when sugar became more available, it was still considered a very precious food item. One can occasionally find in German antique shops silver boxes which were once used as sugar containers. They are fitted with keys.

Sugar has a very interesting history. It is still not known whether the Indians or the Arabs first produced it, but cultivated sugar cane was first found in India by the Greeks under Alexander. In the Middle Ages sugar was brought from the East to Europe via Venice, and then reached England through Germany and Flanders. Columbus was supposed to have taken sugar cane to America, where it was successfully planted. In the sixteenth century sugar cane was brought to Cyprus and Sicily and was cultivated there.

At the beginning of the nineteenth century the German Scientist F. A. Archard found a method of producing sugar from sugar beet. But this discovery was not utilized until the Napoleonic Wars, during which most of Europe was isolated by a British naval blockade from overseas countries and could not import sugar cane. It was then that the production of sugar from beet really started. Today, most European countries use beet sugar.

Since the nineteenth century the production and consumption of sugar has steadily risen. It had only two setbacks (during the two world wars). But during those years of war the incidence of diabetes and other diseases arising from the over-consumption of sugar also decreased. From the standpoint of health, these two setbacks were a blessing. Today, the large consumption of sugar has become a great worry to doctors. Some nutritionists consider sugar to be the main cause of obesity and several degenerative diseases. Some put the blame for the present high incidence of coronary thrombosis entirely on sugar.

Some authors on slimming recommend the total avoidance of sugar- and starch-containing foods. This is advice which is easy to give but hard to follow. It would be impossible for the slimmer to avoid *all* carbohydrates. We can cut down on starches and sugar-containing foods, but we cannot omit them completely.

Why is sugar such a dangerous food? Because it has a high calorie value, contains no bulk, and has no vitamins nor minerals. Some nutritionists call sugar the food with empty calories because it supplies only energy, nothing else.

Sugar has other faults too. It can be habit forming. The more sugar we eat the more we crave for it. If we eat more sugar than we need, the level of sugar in our blood rises. To counteract this the Langerhans Islets (small endocrine glands which are embedded in the Pancreas) release insulin which reduces the amount of blood sugar. But these glands do not always function so precisely that they secrete only as much insulin as is necessary. Sometimes, they produce more. In this event the blood sugar falls below its normal level. In such a situation, a person becomes irritable and hungry, and has to take more sugar to relieve his condition. A vicious circle starts. The more sugar he eats, the more he may need afterwards. But this process cannot go on indefinitely. In time, the Langerhans Islets become exhausted and produce less and less insulin. Finally, they are not even able to supply enough insulin to cope with the normal carbohydrate metabolism. If this happens, the person has reached the state of diabetes.

Hence it is not surprising that during the last two world wars the number of new cases of diabetes fell considerably. With the lower consumption of sugar the incidence of other degenerative diseases also fell.

How can we reduce our high intake of sugar? For many of us, who have become accustomed to sweet drinks and food, it would not now be easy to take them unsweetened. But we have a valuable substitute for sugar which is free of calories and which can be used to sweeten drinks and solid foods. It is saccharine, which was discovered by Fahlberg and Ramsen in 1879, and has since been found to be a safe and useful sweetening agent.

Many overweight people have an aversion to saccharine. They dislike its taste, and claim that they are aware of its presence in drinks and solid foods, even in very small quantities. Personally, I have never found much difference in taste between saccharine and sugar.

Saccharine can easily become unpalatable if it is used the wrong way.

If you put several teaspoonfuls of *sugar* into drinks, they will remain sweet, even if the sugar has reached saturation point and can no longer be dissolved in the fluid. But this is not so with saccharine. The more saccharine you put into drinks, the less sweet they taste, and finally they will acquire a bitter and metallic taste. Many firms produce saccharine tablets which have the sweetening power of one teaspoonful or two lumps of sugar. As long as you are going to use one tablet for your tea or coffee, you should not find them unpleasant. But some people use more than one tablet, hoping by so doing to increase the sweetness of their drinks. However, they achieve the opposite effect.

Another important fact is that saccharine is unsuitable for cooking. It will undergo a chemical breakdown when exposed to heat. This gives a bitter and metallic taste to food cooked with it. So sweeten foods with saccharine only *after* they have been cooked.

Long after saccharine was discovered, other artificial sweeteners were produced but they have not proved to be as safe for health as saccharine. Among them are sodium cyclamate and calcium cyclamate.

In some countries these substances are no longer permitted to be added to manufactured foods. In some ways, these two substances were better than saccharine because they did not decompose during the process of cooking or baking and did not lose their sweet taste. It is unfortunate that they have been found to be hazardous to health.

Saccharine has also often been suspected of being dangerous to health, but thorough observations during the years since its discovery have proved these suspicions unfounded. It was once thought that saccharine was a mental depressant, that it prevented the absorption of some vitamins from the bowels, and that it caused cancer when used for a long time. But investigations proved that saccharine was harmless, even when taken for a very long time. Saccharine is quickly absorbed by the bowels and is also quickly released from the body. Since saccharine does not accumulate in the body, it cannot cause cumulative ill effects. But it should be remembered again that saccharine is a very strong sweetener, and should therefore be used like a very pungent spice. Every good cook knows how quickly a spice can spoil a dish if too much is added. The same applies to saccharine.

Here are some interesting facts about saccharine. In spite of its long use, its sweetening power has still not been fully evaluated. Some authorities state that saccharine is two hundred times as sweet as sugar, others estimate it to be seven hundred times as sweet. Furthermore, saccharine does not taste sweet at all if it is taken in its pure form. If you put a tablet of saccharine on your tongue for a second or two (a most unpleasant sensation), you will notice that it has a very bitter taste. Saccharine tastes sweet only when diluted in plenty of liquid.

All in all, saccharine is an excellent substitute for sugar. It is *free of calories* and can considerably reduce one's intake of sugar if used the right way. Use it whenever possible, and you will soon see a reduction in your weight.

10
"Slimming" Foods and "Slimming" Aids

THERE are many misleading beliefs about foods which are either supposed to be low in calories or are alleged to have the magic power to melt away body fat. These fallacies have been spread for decades by food fads, health magazines and some newspapers, and have often been willingly accepted by people who have tried to slim.

Brown Bread versus White Bread

One fallacy is that brown bread is less fattening than white. There is no scientific proof for this. The calorie value of brown bread and of white bread is about the same.

What, then, is the difference?

White bread can be baked more easily because white flour rises much better than dark flour. White bread is more digestible than brown, and is more suitable for people suffering from certain diseases of the stomach and the bowels. White flour can also be stored more easily, because it contains less fat than dark, and does not become rancid so easily.

Years ago, white bread had the disadvantage of lacking some of the B vitamins, and iron and calcium. But that deficiency has been remedied, a long time ago. Nowadays white bread is specially fortified. White bread contains a smaller amount of protein compared with brown, but that is hardly of any significance.

Food fads are always full of praise for brown bread, but rarely do they mention its disadvantages. One is that it contains phytic acid, a substance which interferes with the absorption of calcium, necessary for the building of the bones.

In 1942 the British Nutritionists, McCance and Widdowson published a paper which showed that phytic acid found in dark bread interfered with calcium absorption. They also made it clear that the action of phytic acid could be counteracted by adding calcium to dark bread.

Nowadays, brown bread is already fortified with calcium, and no adverse effects are noticed.

The old controversy, whether white or brown bread is more nutritious, was solved soon after the Second World War also by McCance and Widdowson in their experiment with German children in the two orphanages of Duisburg and Wuppertal.

At that time, the food rations in Germany were poor. The children in those two orphanages were undernourished and underweight. Their food consisted mainly of soups, vegetables, potatoes, 3 ozs. of milk and a very small amount of animal protein (about 8 grammes). To find out which type of bread was more nutritious, the children in the orphanage of Duisburg were divided into five groups, each group received unlimited quantities of a certain grade of either white or brown bread. They all thrived equally, no matter what type of bread they ate. A year later there was no difference in their state of nutrition. They had all gained in weight. The experiment proved that the meagre German ration which the children had received in addition to their unlimited quantities of bread, was sufficient to supplement all the small deficiencies of either white or brown bread. It was also shown that white bread is highly nutritious and not an empty food as is so often alleged.

Similar experiments were also made in the orphanage of Wuppertal. But here, part of the bread ration was replaced by fat and sugar. Here also the children recovered from their state of undernutrition and gained weight, no matter what sort of bread they ate.

Toast, Crispbreads, "Protein Breads"

Another erroneous view is that toast is less fattening than new bread. If you toast a slice of new bread, you diminish its content of moisture, you change its flavour and texture by altering part of its carbohydrates, but you don't reduce it by one single calorie. If you prefer toast to new bread, eat it by all means, but do not imagine that it is less fattening. The same applies to crispbreads and "protein breads". Crispbreads were originally made with rye, but they also contain wheat now. Don't think that they are of any great help in slimming. They are breads, from which most of the water has been removed. Water has no calorie value. Bread, free from part of its water, has no reduced calorie value.

During the past years "protein breads" have been put on the market. They are supposed to have a slimming effect. Some people have the impression that "protein breads" are free from starch and contain only protein. This, of course, is not true. Only a *small part* of the starch has been replaced by protein in such types of bread; and that small alteration does not greatly alter its calorie value.

There is something else, which many people forget. Bread is rarely eaten dry. It is often taken with fat (butter), marmalade or jam, which may double or treble its calorie content.

Did you say that you only ate a slice or two of bread for breakfast? Don't think that your calorie intake was low if you added butter and marmalade to it.

Margarine versus Butter

There is a popular myth that margarine is lower in calories than butter. The truth is that both contain the same amount of calories. You are not going to save any calories by substituting margarine for butter. It is difficult to find the reason for the misconception. Perhaps it has something to do with the lower price of margarine.

Many people also believe that butter is a food of higher nutritional value than margarine. This was true many years ago, when margarine lacked the two important vitamins A and D. But now margarine is fortified with all the vitamins which are to be found in butter.

There is another reason why so many slimmers substitute margarine for butter. Proportionally with the increase in obesity, there has also been an increase in the incidence of coronary thrombosis. Many nutritionists blame animal fats, which belong to the groups of saturated fats, for the hardening of the arteries. They consider polyunsaturated fats, such as some of the vegetable —and fish oils, as a safer food for avoiding coronary thrombosis. Unfortunately, margarine is not safer than butter. Although it is made from vegetable or fish oils, these oils have been turned into saturated fats when hardened into solid margarine. In short, there is not much difference between butter and margarine in their calorie or nutritional value.

"Sugar Free" Foods

Equally deceptive is the belief that "sugar free" jams, marmalades, chocolates, tinned fruits, etc., are not fattening. The trouble is, however, that the sugar in these foods has been replaced by *sorbitol*. Although sorbitol is less sweet than sugar, it contains the same amount of calories.

Manufactured foods labelled "free from added sugar" may therefore be just as fattening as those made with sugar. For diabetics sorbitol has the advantage over sugar that it is slowly absorbed from the guts and does not raise the level of sugar in the blood so quickly. Diabetics are very sensitive to a sudden rise of sugar in the blood. But sorbitol is useless for slimmers, because ultimately *it is* absorbed and supplies the same amount of calories as sugar.

For the slimmer the only safe sweetening substance which is free from calories is saccharine. We therefore ask why slimming foods are not sweetened with saccharine instead of sorbitol. The reason is that it has no preserving property. Sugar and sorbitol not only sweeten food and improve its taste, they also preserve it. They withdraw the water from micro organisms, and prevent them from flourishing (bacteria are very sensitive to dehydration, and soon die without water). To make "slimming foods" more saleable, some manufacturers have added to them small quantities of saccharine, but they still usually contain either sugar or sorbitol.

It is worthwhile to inspect the labels on such foods. If sorbitol is mentioned among the ingredients you might just as well buy foods prepared with sugar which are equally fattening and less expensive.

Glucose versus Sugar

Glucose is often imagined to be low in calories. It is a dangerous fallacy because glucose has the same calorie content as sugar. What makes the situation worse is that for sweetening tea or coffee, glucose is often taken in far greater quantities than sugar simply because glucose is only half as sweet.

It is wrong to think that foods which do not taste sweet are low in calories. Pears and apples both contain the same amount of sugar. Apples taste less sweet because they have a higher content of malic acid which counteracts the sweetness of sugar. But the calorie value of pears and apples is the same.

Another common fallacy is that glucose supplies more energy than sugar. There are on the market various drinks and tonics which contain glucose for this reason. But sugar, as soon as it reaches the stomach, is split into glucose and fructose and is used by the body in the same way as glucose taken by mouth.

Honey

Some fads never tire of hailing honey for its alleged outstanding qualities. It is supposed to be loaded with vitamins and minerals. Nutritionists are of a different opinion. What does honey actually contain? 20% of it is water. Its chief contents are fruit sugar and glucose (about 76%). It does not contain the important vitamins A and D; it has only traces of some of the B vitamins and vitamin C, and negligible amounts of some minerals.

Honey has not many advantages over table sugar. Its taste may be more pleasant because of its distinctive flavour. Weight for weight its calorie value is a little lower than that of table sugar, because it contains 20% water. But for the slimmer honey is just as dangerous as sugar. After digestion sugar and honey contribute in the same way to the accumulation of body fat if they are eaten in greater quantities than the body requires.

Brown Sugar and Treacle versus White Sugar

Brown sugar and black treacle are not going to help you either, if you want to lose weight. Both are highly favoured in some quarters. Brown sugar is neither more nutritious than white sugar, nor has it fewer calories as some fads claim. It is only a slightly impure sugar and contains a very small amount of minerals.

Black treacle is supposed to be another "miracle stuff", and to supply you with energy without the danger of increasing your weight. Black treacle is a by-product in the making of sugar. Contrary to some claims, its content of iron and calcium is only small. Weight for weight, it has fewer calories than sugar because of its water content (about 28%). But it contains the considerable amount of 67% of invert sugar. If you are going to try to reduce weight with black treacle, you will be unpleasantly surprised.

Lemon Juice

Does lemon juice reduce your weight? This fallacy has been handed down to us through many decades. It is recommended in many slimming diets, but the reason is a mystery. If taken with other food it does not reduce its calorie content, nor has it any effect on the body weight. If you eat a breakfast of e.g. 500 calories, you are not going to reduce it by a single calorie if you add to it lemon juice. Nor does lemon juice "melt away your body fat".

Hot Water

Drinking hot water before breakfast is sometimes suggested. Water has the only advantage that—like lemon juice—it is free of calories, but it won't decrease the calorie value of foods taken with it.

Brown and White Eggs

While we are still at breakfast, let us discuss the old argument over the nutritious value of brown and white eggs. Although it was proved a long time ago that there is no difference in their food value, many people still prefer brown eggs. Slimmers might like to know that the calorie value of white and brown eggs is identical.

Battery Eggs versus Free Range Eggs

Battery eggs have become a great target of food fads, who consider them to be of low nutritional value and lacking the vitamins found in free range eggs. There is no evidence for this claim. Nor is there any calorie difference.

Yoghourt

A food which has been popular for centuries in most Balkan countries, and has later found its way to other countries of Europe and to the United States of America. It came rather late to Britain, and is used here not so much as a food but as a health cure. It is supposed to cure hardening of the arteries, nervous exhaustion, various diseases of the bowels and of the skin, and also obesity. Curiously enough, it is also thought to help thin people to gain weight.

Yoghourt was originally believed to have the power to prevent poisoning of the large bowels by acting against putrefactive bacteria. Later investigations showed no evidence for this view.

What actually is yoghourt? It is milk, which has been fermented under heat by some bacteria such as bacillus bulgaricus, baccillus acidophilus and bacillus bifidus. During the process of fermentation the milk sugar is turned into lactic acid, which gives the milk a slight sour taste and a creamy consistency. But there is no change in the vitamins, minerals and proteins in the milk during that process. Neither does the calorie value of the milk change when turned into yoghourt. In short, if you prefer milk, you will get from it the same nutriments and the same amount of calories as you do from yoghourt.

Unfortunately manufacturers realised a long time ago that some people in Western Countries could not adapt themselves to the taste of yoghourt. They have therefore improved its taste by adding to it sugar and various fruit flavours. Sugar, of course, increases the calorie content of yoghourt and makes it even less suitable than milk for slimming.

Goats' Milk versus Cows' Milk

There is little difference in nutritional or calorie value between cows' or goats' milk. Goats' milk is hard to get in most parts of Britain, although some health stores sell yoghourt made from goats' milk. If you want to slim, the drinking of goats' milk won't decrease your waist line.

Fresh Milk versus Pasteurised Milk

Another fallacy often propagated by quacks is that milk drunk fresh from the cow is more wholesome than if pasteurised. It is a dangerous misconception, because milk is not only an excellent food for human beings, but also for germs. The decrease of tuberculosis in many Western countries during the past decades is mainly due to the sale of pasteurised milk. Pasteurisation kills all the dangerous germs. During the process of heating, the protein and calcium content of the milk remains intact. (Part of the vitamins C and B are destroyed, but that is not significant, because they can easily be obtained from other foods). The calorie value of the milk does not alter after pasteurisation.

"Slimming Foods"—How Good are They?

The number of manufactured slimming foods has multiplied in recent years. These are expensive and of little use to those who want to keep their weight down permanently. Various brands of slimming biscuits (crackers in America), slimming powders, fruit drinks and candies are now exhibited which are supposed to melt away the superfluous fat in a very short time. In the advertisement columns of magazines and newspapers are shown photographs of people who have undergone cures with such wonder-foods and have turned their fat and unsightly body shapes into sylph-like figures. No doubt a few have been successful with that type of treatment, but you won't find in the same papers the photographs of thousands of other people, who had started the same type of treatment, but had not been able to continue it, because of its monotonous regimen and severity. The biscuits and powders are mostly unbalanced foods with little roughage and may cause severe constipation. Apart from these defects, they never teach you sensible ways of eating. If you are one of those heroes who have been able to shed all those superfluous pounds with those miracle foods, you have still not learned how to retain your normal weight afterwards, because you cannot live forever on biscuits and powders.

Preserved Foods versus Fresh Foods

Many people are convinced that canned or frozen foods have a lower nutritional value than fresh ones.

Careful investigations have proved that only a few nutriments are lost during the process of food preservations. Some vitamins became lost during the heating operations, but the same happens when food is cooked. Nevertheless, only very few people in this country suffer from lack of vitamins, because we also eat other types of foods which supply us with plenty.

Other important constituents of food, such as carbohydrates, proteins and fats are not destroyed during the process of canning or freezing.

Food preservation has been practised for many centuries. Salt and vinegar were probably the first preservatives. Later, when sugar became more widely available and cheap, it was also used for preserving some foods, such as fruit. Smoking of some foods, such as meat and fish, is an old method of conservation.

Some people consider that additives such as dyes, which are often used during the process of preservation, are poisons, but no health authority would permit their use if they were detrimental to health. It is not the fault of the manufacturers that some of the canned foods have to be dyed. People would not buy them otherwise. Who would purchase greyish-green looking peas in cans? But that is their normal colour after heating. A bright green dye has to be added to make peas look more "natural". Strawberries, after heating, look brown, but that colour does not appeal to the customer. They have to be bright red. No wonder then that a red dye has to be added to make them saleable. The same applies to tomato soup. Nobody would buy the normal reddish-grey tomato soup. It has to be glowing red.

Preserved foods have many advantages. A great variety is now available all the year round. Preserved foods are also safeguarded from dangerous bacteria and moulds. They are more suitable for transport over long distances. Many countries which suffered in the past from seasonal starvation benefit today from the import of preserved food.

Some canned and frozen foods are very useful for the slimmer, especially low calorie vegetables, fish and meat. But there are also preserved foods which are taboo for the slimmer, for example, canned fruit which should be avoided because of its high calorie content. During the process of canning, syrup is added to the fruit and it absorbs a considerable quantity of sugar. The more concentrated the syrup, the more sugar. Even if you tried to eat the fruit without syrup, you would still consume a considerable amount of sugar. A look at the labels of such tins will show you that they contain either "syrup", "heavy syrup", or "extra heavy syrup". Whatever the concentration may be, keep away from canned fruit, if you want to reduce your weight.

Wonder Foods

Apart from claims about the magic qualities of honey and yoghourt, similar assertions are made about wheat germ, yeast, royal jelly, safflower oil, biochemic salt, etc. Some food fads do not consider them as aids for slimming, but as essentials for general health. Many of these items have, however, already found their place on shelves for slimming foods in chemists' shops and health stores.

These "magic" foods are not going to reduce an ounce of your weight if you add them to your ordinary daily meals. Nor do they have the property of melting away your fat or of preventing you from gaining weight if your intake of calories is greater than your requirements.

Factory-Reared Meat Foods

Another hotly discussed subject is meat from animals which have been reared with the help of antibiotics and hormones. Some people aver that such meat lacks nutritional value and may even cause cancer. None of these claims has been proved so far. The use of hormones and antibiotics has accelerated the growth of some domestic animals, such as chickens, turkeys, calves, pigs, etc., and has made their meat cheaper and more plentiful for the less wealthy. Chickens e.g. which were once expensive, can now be bought by people of slender means. For the slimmer, the present broiler chickens are more suitable than the old type of fowl because they contain less fat.

Many people are sure that today's chickens are inferior in taste to those they had years ago. But we have often heard similar statements about manufactured foods, which are nowadays prepared the same way as they were years ago, and are no longer "as good" as before. There is, of course, some truth in these statements. As we grow older, food does not taste so good as in our younger days because the number of taste buds on the tongue decreases with age. Nevertheless, I personally still prefer today's broiler chickens to those drenched with fat which I ate years ago.

Vegetarian Diets

A vegetarian diet is not always the right way to a slim figure. Admittedly, some of the low calorie vegetables are a boon to the slimmer, but not all foods derived from plants have a low calorie value. Sugar and flour, two of the main causes of obesity, are vegetable products. The calorie value of vegetable margarines is not lower than that of margarine containing animal fat.

Pure vegetarian food has also some disadvantages. Vegetarians can tell us that many strong animals live entirely on vegetarian foods. But the human body is not able to utilise vegetarian food to the same extent as the bodies of plant-eating animals. Ruminants, horses, pigs, rabbits, etc., can even turn straw into energy, something which the human intestines are not able to do.

There are some vegetarians who only eat small amounts of bulk, but consume great quantities of liquidated vegetarian foods. This way of eating is of little use to the slimmer. Liquids do not remain for very long in the stomach and do not make you feel full for any length of time. Moreover, the lack of bulk may cause severe constipation.

Vegetable protein is also of lower quality than animal

protein. It is usually mixed with starch and fibres and is less easily digestible. Fortunately, most vegetarians do not confine themselves to foods which are derived entirely from plants, but also eat some animal foods such as eggs, milk and cheese. In this way they consume proteins of very high quality.

Vegetarian food also lacks the important vitamin B 12. The absence of this vitamin may cause anaemia and some disturbances of the central nervous system. In short, a strictly vegetarian diet is not the ideal way to a slim figure.

"Slimming Aids"

Apart from "magic foods", other slimming helps have become fashionable in the past years.

It is sad to see that a number of people, after unsuccessful slimming attempts, take resort in various "slimming" devices which are advertised. "Reducing" ointments, creams and lotions, bath salts, elastic corsets, rubber garments and exercise machines are some of these "slimming" helps. They are of no value to the slimmer.

"Reducing" ointments, creams and lotions do not melt away your fat, because they never penetrate the skin and do not reach the underlying fat tissue. Neither would they have any effect on your weight even if they reached the fat tissue. So far, no substance has been found which would reduce the amount of fat by direct contact with it.

"Reducing" bath salts are another useless item for the slimmer. They consist mainly of Epsom salt or bicarbonate of soda with added perfume. There is not the slightest proof that these bath salts have any effect on the body fat.

Neither do Turkish or Sauna baths reduce one's body fat. They only cause a temporary loss of body water by profuse sweating. People weigh less after such baths, but they have lost only water and not fat. They are usually so thirsty afterwards that they have to drink excessive amounts of water to quench their thirst. By so doing, they regain their lost weight. It should also be mentioned that Turkish baths are not always harmless. They can even be dangerous for people who suffer from a weak heart or high blood pressure.

Appliances which are supposed to slim your figure are elastic corsets and rubber or plastic garments. They will never strip away your fat. These garments are uncomfortable and unhygienic, especially on hot days, and they are useless for those who want to lose weight.

Other devices are exercise machines and slimming gadgets. People spend a lot of money to have their bodies shaken and massaged with all sorts of vibrating machines, but they never lose weight except by dieting simultaneously. Advertisers sell various sorts of rubber rollers which are supposed to roll away the surplus fat. No effect on weight has been noticed with these gadgets, though there can be the beneficial effect of strengthening the abdominal muscles, which may improve the figure.

11
Should We Believe the Advertisements?

MANUFACTURERS of slimming aids have ways to persuade people which are forbidden to the medical profession. They are allowed to advertise and to produce publicly testimonials from patients. Doctors are debarred from such methods.

A manufacturer of some unscientific remedy can show in his advertisements testimonials from celebrities or from ordinary people, who, after their first attempt with such remedies, are genuinely convinced that these have done the trick. But when these patients, after further weeks of trying, find that the remedies have not fulfilled their promise, they rarely inform the producer about this failure. Even if the manufacturer were to receive letters of complaints, would he publish them?

Then consider the psychological effect of ordinary food advertising. Take, for instance, advertisements for chocolates which we notice on television. We see a slim and glamorous model, holding a box of chocolates, who gets into a state of ecstasy when she puts a piece of chocolate into her mouth. There is nothing misleading in that advertisement, but overweight people may come to the conclusion that chocolate is not as fattening as it is supposed to be. If a slim and pretty girl can eat it, why should it be bad for me? But that slim model probably never touches chocolate outside the television studio.

The same applies to similar advertisements shown on hoardings and in magazines. No matter how fattening the food is, a nubile girl is a must for publicising it.

Even magazines on slimming are not always free from misleading advertisements. We often find in such periodicals articles on slimming which have been written by authors of high repute. We also find there many useful cooking recipes.

But what use is it to have the sound advice of the articles, if the advertisements in the same paper tell us to do the opposite? People with some knowledge of nutrition can soon sort out the useful articles from the misleading advertisements, but others have difficulty in separating the wheat from the chaff. They may even consider the advertisements just as useful as the articles from reputable authors on slimming.

What do we find among these advertisements? Candies which are supposed to melt away the body fat in a short time, several brands of bread which are claimed by the producers to be of great help in slimming, but vary only little in their calorie value from ordinary bread. We see coloured photographs of the most mouth watering chocolates, chocolate biscuits, and various other biscuits which are regarded as great aids in slimming. A dairy firm displays among different dairy products a carton of double cream which no doctor would dare to prescribe for the slimmer. Several types of "slimming" garments are never absent from those advertisements. We even find the advertisement of an astrologist who tries to convince us that out diets depend on our stars.

Advertisements need not be useless. They may even be of great value. Those who remember the war and post-war years look back with gratitude upon the frequent infor-

SHOULD WE BELIEVE THE ADVERTISEMENTS? 79

mation which we used to receive from the then Ministry of Food. When some foods were scarce or unobtainable, we were given helpful advice about others of equal nutritional value. Housewives and caterers will remember the many useful cooking recipes which were issued in those days.

Today, when the health of the nation is jeopardised by increasing obesity, and the incidence of diseases due to it is steadily rising, advertisements of a similar nature as those issued during the time of emergency would be a blessing to the nation. Perhaps the day will come when the Ministry of Health will supply information about our nutritional needs just as the Ministry of Food did during wartime.

12
Do Vitamins Help?

IF you take a look in the "slimming department" of chemists' shops or health stores, or watch their window displays of slimming articles, you will rarely miss vitamin tablets. You will also find manufactured foods fortified with vitamins.

Many slimmers think that vitamins are a must for reducing weight, but the truth is that they are completely useless. Extensive research has proved that there is not a shred of evidence that any of the vitamins has any effect upon weight. The addition of vitamins to a high calorie diet decreases neither its calorie content, nor the accumulated fat in the body. A sensible reducing diet does not require extra vitamins, because it *already contains* all the vitamins necessary for the body.

It is surprising that so many people still take large amounts of vitamins, although vitamin deficiency has nearly disappeared from most Western countries. Nowadays, more patients are in hospital with an overdose of vitamins than from lack of them.

Vitamins are certainly of great importance to the body, but this does not mean that we have to take more than we need. Some of the vitamins may even cause great bodily harm if taken in excess.

It was a great event in the history of medicine when the first vitamin was discovered in 1912. Since then progress has been made in the discovery of further vitamins. Most

DO VITAMINS HELP?

diseases due to vitamin deficiency can now be cured. The most notable examples are Scurvy, Beri-Beri and Rickets although it would take many pages to describe in detail all the vitamins which have been discovered so far. Readers who are interested in this subject should consult specialist works.

As this book deals mainly with the subject of slimming, it is sufficient to emphasize that none of the numerous vitamins discovered so far has any effect on the reduction of body weight.

One important fact should be mentioned to those who are enthusiastic about vitamin pills. An overdose of some of the vitamins, especially of the fat-soluble vitamins A and D, may cause severe bodily harm.

The body cannot eliminate superfluous vitamin A quickly. An increased amount of vitamin A in the body can cause damage to the bones, skin, liver and various other organs. Children given an excess of vitamin A, complain of loss of appetite, sickness, itching of the skin, pain in the bones and other symptoms.

It is interesting that a long time ago Eskimos learned from experience to avoid eating the liver of polar bears which has a very large content of vitamin A. Diseases due to lack of vitamin A, however, are hardly known in Western countries.

An overdose of vitamin D may also cause severe damage to the body. It may lead to increased calcium deposits in the large blood vessels, the heart, kidneys, lungs and other organs. People suffering from an excess of vitamin D in their body complain of loss of appetite, sickness, fatigue and frequent urination owing to damage to their kidneys.

An excessive intake of the vitamins of the B complex and vitamin C, has fortunately, little effect on the body, because these vitamins are soluble in water and can easily be expelled from the body through the kidneys. This is a blessing for the ardent followers of some quacks and food fads who never tire of advising us to take an additional supply of the vitamins B and C in our daily diet.

Vitamins are of great importance to the body. Several diseases caused by lack of vitamins have now been cured. But this fact does not mean that we have to take more vitamins than we need. They will not reduce our weight.

13
Do Drugs Help?

*"I firmly believe that if the whole
materia medica, as now used, could
be sunk to the bottom of the sea, it
would be all the better for mankind—
And all the worse for the fishes."*
　　　　　Oliver Wendel Holmes, 1842.

MEDICINE has made great progress since the end of the last century. A detailed account of all the useful drugs which have been introduced during the past decades would fill a heavy volume. A mere outline of all those drugs would take many pages.

The discovery of hormones and vitamins, the successful administration of diphtheria antitoxin, the introduction of the preparation Salvarsan by Paul Ehrlich for treating syphilis, the discovery of Insulin by Banting and Best as a remedy for diabetes, Minot's and Murphy's use of liver as a specific treatment for pernicious anaemia (a treatment later improved by vitamin B 12), Domagk's introduction of Sulphonamide and Fleming's discovery of Penicillin as a cure for most infectious diseases, these are only a few of the great landmarks in medicine since 1900.

This century has also seen the introduction of many useful and lifesaving drugs, such as pain relieving remedies, drugs for metal poisoning, streptomycin, the specific preparation for tuberculosis and so on.

Oliver Wendel Holmes, the 19th century doctor and philosopher would have revised his opinion about the uselessness of drugs, had he been alive today. But his belief that medicines are only fit to be dumped into the sea is still valid for most of the slimming drugs. There are still no drugs which can melt away superfluous fat in spite of the many claims made by manufacturers.

Some of the slimming drugs can at best be used as "crutches" at the beginning of a slimming cure. At present, there exists no medicine which can reduce weight without simultaneous dieting.

After the discovery of so many miracle drugs during the past decades, research workers have not been idle in seeking a suitable drug for slimming too. So far, however, they have met with no success, in spite of hard work.

A suitable medicine for weight reducing would solve many problems. We live at a time when overweight is even more dangerous that it was years ago when life expectation was lower. After the age of forty we become more susceptible to degenerative diseases caused by overweight. Not that young people suffer less from overweight than older ones. A doctor could tell many heartbreaking stories of youthful patients who would have given anything to lose their superfluous fat. "The jolly fat man" is a figment of the imagination. I have never found that fat people are jolly in a surgery or clinic.

Which, then, are the slimming drugs that are commonly used?

Appetite Suppressing Drugs

The great majority of overweight people take appetite-suppressing drugs. This medicine became popular in the forties, although the first experiment with it was made in 1938. The first appetite-suppressing preparations belonged chemically to the group of Amphetamines; later, drugs of other chemical compositions, but with similar effects, appeared on the market.

At first, it appeared that these drugs were suitable remedies. They were praised equally by the medical and lay press. But during the course of years, disadvantages were found. First, it was noted that the appetite-suppressing effect wore off after two or three months, sometimes even earlier. It was noticed, moreover, that these tablets were of little use if the diet was not restricted at the same time. In the long run, it did not matter whether people took these tablets or not. They lost an equal amount of weight with or without tablets as long as they controlled their diet.

Apart from the short duration of their appetite-suppressing property, many of these drugs, when used for long periods, showed dangerous side effects. Some caused loss of sleep, irritability, restlessness and even addiction. Others caused dizziness, rapid beating of the heart, increased blood pressure, sweating, blurred vision, vomiting or constipation. A few of these drugs were dangerous for people who suffered from narrow blood vessels of the heart and from high blood pressure.

Extracts of the Thyroid Gland

Many years before the appetite-suppressing drugs were known, doctors used extracts of the thyroid gland for the treatment of obesity. This treatment is still used today, more in Europe than in Britain.

One of the main functions of the thyroid gland is to stimulate metabolism. It was therefore thought that the hormone of the thyroid gland would also accelerate the turnover of fat tissue in the human body and help to reduce body weight. But this treatment did not prove effective. It was observed a long time ago that ordinary doses of the thyroid extract were of no use for obese people whose thyroid gland functioned normally. Some specialists on the Continent therefore tried to give higher doses in order to stimulate the metabolism of fat people. Sometimes, these doses were so high that they caused toxic symptoms such as rapid beating of the heart, nervousness, irritability, shaking of the upper limbs and severe sweating. It was also dangerous for conditions of constricted blood vessels of the heart and in diabetes. In spite of all these disadvantages, some obese people are still treated today with the extract of the thyroid gland, without encouraging results.

Some Other Hormones

Other hormones have also been used in the treatment of obesity. They were all expected to stimulate the metabolism of the fat tissue of the body. Among them were the hormones of the front lobe of the hypophysis (a small two-lobed gland at the base of the brain), of the male and female sex glands and of several other glands. But they all proved to be ineffective. Without dietary control no reduction of weight was achieved.

Diuretics

The erroneous belief that water and salt are fattening has already been dealt with in Chapter 5. To reduce the amount of fluid in the body, diuretics are sometimes given to overweight people but they are only effective in patients who suffer from an accumulation of water in their body due to heart failure. Even to such patients, diuretics have to be given with care.

Laxatives

Laxatives are still sometimes prescribed by doctors with the idea that they stimulate the bowels into greater activity, eliminate the food more quickly than usual from the body than under ordinary conditions, and prevent the normal absorption of food. But this is not the right way to lose weight. Sooner or later the bowels will rebel against such ill-treatment.

Laxatives are often taken on the quite erroneous assumption that weight reducing causes constipation. What usually happens is that people often cut down their normal amount of food whilst slimming, so supplying the bowels with little bulk. It is obvious that the amount of stool and the frequency of its evacuation diminishes if there is little bulk in the bowels. Were the slimmer to eat more low calorie vegetables such as cabbage, cauliflower, brussels sprouts, carrots, etc., he would not suffer from constipation. Sensible dieting is a better way of losing weight than taking laxatives.

Hypoglycaemic Drugs

In recent years a number of people have been treated with so-called 'hypoglycaemic' drugs. These drugs, taken orally, have the property of reducing the amount of sugar in the blood. They were first used for overweight diabetics and then tried out on fat people with normal sugar levels in their blood. The results of this treatment have not been very reassuring, although some doctors claim that hypoglycaemic drugs are better than most other preparations for slimming.

Methylcellulose

This is a more harmless remedy which has been used for some years. It contains no active agent, and has therefore no effect on the central nervous system, the heart, blood vessels or any other organ. Because of this it cannot really be termed a drug at all. Nevertheless, it is used as a treatment for obesity because it has the property of swelling when water is added to it, and it is therefore supposed to make you feel full by supplying the stomach with bulk.

Some people claim that methylcellulose swells to ten times its original volume when taken with water. I myself have not found it swelled this much, nor did it make me feel as full as they claim. I put a teaspoonful of this powder into a glass of water and waited for twelve hours. After draining off the water, I found that the volume remaining was about a dessertspoonful. But it may be that even a small quantity of swelled methylcellulose acts differently from food. Because of its jelly-like consistency after absorption of water, it may stick to the inner walls of the stomach and bowels and remain there longer than other foods. There have been reports in medical papers that methylcellulose has been found lying at the narrow parts of the stomach for a considerable time and even perforation of the bowels has been reported.

Originally, methylcellulose came as a powder. Later some manufacturers moulded it into large tablets in order to give it the appearance of a drug. Today, it is also included in some types of "slimming biscuits" and other slimming foods. Whichever way it is taken, it has not done much to reduce the high incidence of obesity.

More Drastic Treatment

In order to lose weight quickly, some people have been willing to undergo some very drastic treatment.

We saw in Chapter 3 that fever increases the energy expenditure of the body, and that more body fat is burned under a raised temperature than under a normal one. Besides, fever also diminishes the appetite so that less food is eaten. Some specialists have therefore attempted to reduce weight by inducing artificial fever. They injected into the patient either small quantities of milk or other substances containing protein, and caused a rise in the patient's body temperature. This treatment gave far from satisfactory results and was soon abandoned.

Another most unpleasant treatment was the use of drugs which caused nausea and vomiting. After taking such preparations, patients were hardly able to eat and lost weight at the expense of their health. These treatments are no longer used today.

One of the most drastic treatments used for obesity was not a drug, but a mutilating operation of the bowels. By connecting the upper part of the small bowels with the large bowel, a considerable part of the small bowels was prevented from functioning so that the body could not utilize all the food which was eaten.

How desperate must those obese people have felt who consented to such a severe treatment in order to lose weight! If they had known more about ways of sensible dieting, they could have lost all their overweight without undergoing such ordeals.

What Quacks Offer You

Apart from slimming 'drugs' which can be obtained on prescription, there are also available a great number of "slimming" medicines which can be bought over the counter.

Many of these preparations contain laxatives, vitamins or methylcellulose. Also on sale are slimming "herbs" or slimming "teas" which are often marketed under oriental names, but contain hardly anything else but a mild laxative.

Some manufacturers offer combinations of drugs in different colours which are supposed to be taken at different times of day. They usually contain vitamins and laxatives. These tablets are often expensive; they may cost pounds.

Occasionally people do lose weight with these preparations. The manufacturers often include sheets of low calorie diets in the packets of their drugs and advise the slimmer to adhere to these diets. There is a small number of people who actually follow these directions. Their loss of weight is due to the diets and not to the tablets.

You will find tablets advertised which are supposed to reduce your weight without the need to diet. "With these tablets you may eat as much as you like and whatever you like and you will lose weight", promise their advertisers. Do not believe them. So far there just does not exist a drug which can reduce your weight without a diet. If there did, there would be no need to advertise it, and the proprietor would become a millionaire overnight.

It is interesting that there are quacks who always claim a 100% cure with their drugs. Their medicines never seem to fail. It is different with the claims of doctors. If a doctor tests a new drug, he makes careful observations on its effect, and then publishes the results of his investigations. Often, the effects of some drugs which showed great promise at first, turn out to be disappointingly poor. Frequently they are no better than medicines which have been used for many years.

Future Slimming Drugs

What new slimming drugs will the future bring forth? It is difficult to say. Whether there will ever be found a safe and effective drug which will increase the fat metabolism or suppress appetite for long periods, without causing side effects, remains to be seen.

In the meantime, be sceptical about newly discovered slimming drugs which are supposed to have all the qualities of safe weight reducing. For more than thirty years I have read articles in medical journals and in the lay press about newly-discovered slimming drugs. Many of these were at first thought to be miraculous but were soon forgotten. Some even turned out to be dangerous after months or years of trial. It is always safer to wait. It takes years to evaluate the effect and safety of a drug.

So far there exists no drug which can replace a diet. It is therefore best to avoid all the present slimming drugs, and to pay more attention to a diet.

14
Unsound and Ineffective Slimming Methods

The High Failure Rate

Doctors are generally fairly conservative when advising on slimming methods. They usually suggest diets of about 1,000 calories per day. Unfortunately, as a result of this only a very small minority of slimmers lose their overweight for good. According to the reports of some American clinics, only 4 per cent of their patients remain permanently slim. Some patients did not even start the treatment recommended by these clinics, others gave up dieting after an initial attempt, a small percentage continued the diet until they had lost all their overweight, but most of these regained their old weight after some time.

Four per cent is a depressingly low figure! No one would undergo an operation, unless it were a life saving one, if he knew that the chance of complete recovery would be only 4 per cent.

The results of treatments suggested by laymen are probably even poorer, although no figures are available for them.

Factors to be Considered

(a) *Amount of Overweight*

Why do some people fail to lose weight? Because they

UNSOUND AND INEFFECTIVE SLIMMING METHODS

are rarely considered as individuals when they receive slimming instructions. Whether the would-be slimmer is 10 or 40 lbs. overweight, whether he is 16 or 60 years old, whether he is a labourer or a sedentary worker, the treatment advised is the same. If these people consult their family doctors they will usually be given a diet sheet in the range of 1,000 calories daily. If they take advice from some books, magazines or newspapers, they will often be told to follow some bizarre low calorie diets, sometimes as low as 600 calories per day. Are these very low calorie diets always justified? Take, for example, a woman whose weight at the age of twenty was normal, but who gradually gained 10 lbs. in weight by the time she was thirty.

A gain of 10 lbs. during 10 years is not very much. She must have eaten very little above her daily requirement. Does she need to adopt a crash diet of 600 calories a day in order to lose her superfluous 10 lbs.? Is it necessary for her to alter all her meals and to change her eating habits drastically in order to reduce her moderate overweight? Of course not. One single alteration in her daily food intake would probably be sufficient to reduce her weight gradually and to keep it normal for good. Which food item she has to omit depends on her eating habits. If she is used to having a pudding with one of her meals, she must either omit it or replace it by another food of low calorie value such as fresh fruit. Perhaps she is accustomed to high calorie snacks such as sandwiches, cakes, biscuits, chocolates between meals or during the evening hours. The omission of one of these snacks is all that would be necessary. Perhaps she drinks daily several cups of tea or coffee, sweetened with sugar. Then the substitution of saccharine for sugar would be enough. But need she adopt the same diet that is given to a woman of 40 lbs. overweight? Obviously not!

(b) *Age*

What is the difference between the calorie requirement of a youth of 16 and a man of 60? At the age of 16 a man has reached the peak of his calorie requirement. He may need between 3,000 and 4,000 calories per day. But a man of 60 may need only 2,000 calories per day. Therefore on a 2,000 or even higher calorie diet the young man of 16 would probably lose the same amount as the man of 60 would lose on a 1,000 calorie diet. But doctors tend to give them both identical diet sheets.

(c) *Occupation*

Let us look at a third example: two men with an overweight of 30 lbs. One is a labourer performing heavy manual work, the other is a clerk in a sedentary occupation. Even if both are of the same size and of the same age, they do not need the same diet. Yet here again both will be given the same diet sheets. The labourer will lose more weight than the clerk during the same period because his energy expenditure is greater.

(d) *National Eating Habits and Financial Circumstances*

Doctors give too little consideration to eating habits and to slimmers' means. People differ as individuals. Likes and dislikes of foods must not be ignored.

Individuals and even nations find it very hard to accept new eating habits, even if on the point of starvation. Some could not change their eating habits at all. A classical example is the observation made in 1943 in Bengal where famine was raging because of the failure of the rice crop. The U.S.A. sent large quantities of wheat to Bengal, but the Bengalese were not able to eat it. They starved rather than eat wheat which they had never tasted previously.

Those who remember the war and post-war years in Great Britain will recall some of the new foods which were brought here from America such as Spam (canned meat), dried eggs, dehydrated potatoes, etc. But as soon as the emergency ended, and the customary British foods became more widely available, people returned to their old eating habits.

While food scarcity still existed several attempts were made to encourage people to eat new types of foods. Whale-meat was one. The prevailing shortage of meat seemed to provide a suitable occasion to introduce this. But it never caught on, although some people did try to eat it. When beef, lamb and pork were again available in their former quantities, whale-meat was quickly forgotten.

It is therefore unwise to tell an overweight foreigner, recently settled in this country, to adapt himself to a low calorie British diet. It would be futile to persuade a Frenchman to omit bread completely. It could be possible to induce a Frenchman to cut down on bread, but useless to tell him not to eat bread at all. It would be just as hopeless to tell an Italian to stop eating spaghetti.

Crash Diets

Although it has long been known that eating habits cannot be changed quickly, little consideration has been given to this in working out diets. Slimmers are often advised not only to alter all their eating habits abruptly, but also to reduce their total intake so much that these diets, called 'crash diets' would be better named starvation diets. Advisers of such crash diets have little knowledge of calorie values and less of human nature.

In some crash diets even portions of low calorie foods which could not have harmed the slimmer are unnecessarily reduced. In one diet sheet the number of lettuce leaves for a salad was limited to three, in another, only six slices of cucumber were permitted. A third diet advised the slimmer to eat only one small tomato with his meal; a fourth allowed only four small radishes in a salad.

This is senseless. One can eat plenty of lettuce, cucumber, tomatoes or radishes without danger of gaining weight. Lettuce and cucumber each contain only 3 calories per ounce, or 48 calories per pound. Tomatoes and radishes contain 4 calories per ounce (64 calories per pound), an insignificant number for such a large weight of food. Why the slimmer should limit himself to one small tomato is more than puzzling. It would not matter if he were to add 3 or 4 tomatoes to his salad.

Most slimmers carry on with their usual occupations while they are on a crash diet. How can one expect an overweight manual labourer, who has been accustomed to consuming 5,000 or even more calories per day, to become suddenly used to a 600 calorie diet and to continue his daily toil? Even a sedentary worker could not carry on with such a diet without feeling hungry.

Oddly enough, most advocates of such diets assure the slimmers that they are not going to be hungry when following these diets. My experience was quite different when I tried to follow a crash diet many years ago. I was very hungry and I had to give up after a few days. Several of my patients have had the same experience.

Overweight people are told that they are not going to be hungry when dieting, because the body has enough reserves (in the form of fat) on which to draw when energy is required. But our body cannot be compared with a larder which supplies us with food without causing any inconvenience. When the stomach is empty, we experience unpleasant hunger pangs, no matter how much superfluous fat there is around. We have read in an earlier chapter (see Chapter 7) that under special circumstances an empty stomach does not make us feel hungry. We are not usually hungry when we get up early in the morning or after fasting for several days. Neither are we hungry on an empty stomach when we are in a state of anxiety or fear. But in ordinary circumstances we do have very unpleasant hunger sensations on an empty stomach.

There are, of course, always a few heroes (or heroines!) who have been able to endure crash diets for some weeks. But will they have benefited? Yes, they will have lost a lot of weight in a short time. But they cannot live on a crash diet forever. Because they have not learned to eat sensibly, they will later resume their old eating habits and gradually regain their old weight, which they have briefly lost so heroically. Would it not have been better to acquire sensible permanent eating habits, even if it had taken longer? The omission of their daily pudding, the substitution of plain boiled potatoes for chips, of saccharine for sugar or perhaps a daily reduction in bread—these would have taught them permanent good eating habits. The weight loss on a diet such as this might not have been quick, but it would have been effective and persistent.

Health Farms

People who have found it difficult to maintain crash diets at home and who have ample means to pay for starvation diets in luxurious surroundings, have for some time taken refuge in "Health Farms". In such places one can lose a great amount of weight, without being tortured by the sight of high calorie foods. Weight losses of up to 10 lbs. per week are not uncommon. Yes, people lose a lot of weight in Health Farms, but they gain it just as quickly once they are back home again.

It is, perhaps, not surprising that guests at such Health Farms lose so much weight so quickly, because they are not only put on near-starvation diets but also deprived of sufficient water. Salt is often completely omitted. Some residents report that they suffer more from thirst than from hunger. One female reporter, who was a guest in such a place, told of a man who was so tortured by hunger that he ate half a grapefruit, served for breakfast, *together with the skin.*

This treatment is certainly not a satisfactory way to teach overweight people proper eating habits. We can take it for granted that the hungry man we have mentioned did not eat grapefruit with the skin again. As he had not learned sensible eating habits, he probably resumed his old bad ones.

The same reporter mentioned other guests, who, after days of starvation could no longer tolerate this situation and occasionally left the place to have a proper meal outside.

It would be much better if slimmers in such institutions were made to learn right eating habits. They could be given attractive low calorie foods, but not so low in calories as to create intense hunger. They could also be served with larger portions of low calorie foods. The restriction of water and the omission of salt are completely unnecessary.

Can we entirely blame the managements of these Health Farms for their very strict and unscientific diets? No! It is unfortunately an old desire of overweight people to lose their excessive weight quickly.

Health Farms would be less well patronised if their guests left them with a loss of only one or two pounds in weight in a week.

Total Starvation

Encouraged by observations on human beings who had starved for days or weeks without experiencing hunger, some nutritionists started to use similar starvation treatments on fat people in 1959. These were first tried out in the U.S.A. and then used in other countries.

These treatments were undertaken only in hospitals under strict medical supervision. The patients received only water and vitamins. Nothing else was given to them, not even foods of the lowest calorie value.

The resulting weight losses from such treatments were far greater than those from crash or semi-starvation diets. In the beginning, some people lost between 2 and 8 pounds daily. But when the patients became lighter the weight losses gradually dropped to 1 pound daily. It was obvious that the initial loss of weight was not so much of fat as of water. As the patients were deprived of salt, the water was quickly drained away from the body.

At first, this total starvation treatment looked very promising. It enabled some very fat people to lose weight very quickly. But soon several disadvantages became apparent. Some patients began to suffer from diseases of the bowels such as ulcerative colitis. Deaths due to heart attacks have also been reported after such total starvation treatments.

The long-term effects after extensive fasting were not much better than those after crash diets or semi-starvation diets. Patients had learned very little about how to retain their new weight after such a rigid treatment. Most of the slimmers resumed their old eating habits and eventually regained their previous weights.

1,000 Calorie Diets

Diets which are mainly used in hospitals, in obesity clinics and by family doctors are the '1,000 calorie' diets.

These are better endured than the severe rigid diets but they also have unsatisfactory permanent results.

What are the disadvantages of these diets, apart from their poor long term effects? They are not applied individually to people. Some slimmers do not need such low calorie diets. They could easily slim on a higher calorie diet. Some would benefit—as we have seen already—from only a single alteration in their daily food intake.

But can the doctor be blamed for supplying every slimmer with the same diet sheet? Certainly not! A doctor's time nowadays is very limited. It would take him hours to ascertain particulars of the eating habits of each individual patient. It would also take him a considerable time to give advice about an individual diet and to give to each patient details of what special foods to take. It is even questionable whether a doctor would be able to find out all the bad eating habits of his patients.

Single-Item Diets

A number of single-item diets have been (and still are being) suggested to slimmers.

One such was the potato diet. But to eat day after day, even for only a few weeks, nothing but potatoes for breakfast, lunch and supper must be a great ordeal.

Other diets were the milk diets, the banana diets, apple diets, etc. On the Continent, a vegetable and fruit juice diet has often been advised for reducing weight. Some writers have been eager to persuade slimmers to go on a pure- or high-protein diet. This diet is very difficult to follow, because it can easily become repugnant. A large amount of protein eaten daily may also cause strain on the kidneys.

Since the intake of fat has been considered not to cause any gain in body weight(!) one author suggested eating nothing but fat steak three times daily.

Manufacturers have not been idle in compiling diets of depressing monotony. Some years ago one firm started producing a powder which contained protein among a few other ingredients. Slimmers were asked to take a particular amount of this powder, diluted with water four times daily. This daily dose of powder contained 900 calories. Ask yourself how long you could carry on with such a monotonous diet or what the long term benefits would be, if you did manage to endure it.

Nutritionists have long known that some foods can be eaten daily without becoming distasteful, as long as they are taken together with other foods. In most European countries, bread, potatoes and beef are eaten daily, mixed up with other foods. But they could not be eaten singly. In Far Eastern countries, rice is a food which is eaten daily. But even the poorest Asiatic could not live for very long on rice alone. He has to add some other foods to make the rice palatable. The same applies to spaghetti which is eaten daily by the Italians. Most of us dislike eating the same type of meal daily. Cooks in institutions have always known that it is disastrous to serve their inmates with the same menus for only two days in succession. Even a family frowns at the housewife who serves the same meal for several days.

It is surprising that some experts on slimming completely ignore these points and persist in advising slimmers to adhere to the most monotonous diets. The slimmer will never learn to eat properly if he follows such regimes.

There are other diets which do not appear to be as monotonous as single-item diets. One such is the "Hay" diet which permits the slimmer to eat alternately proteins and carbohydrates, but never together. Strict adherence to such diets is almost impossible because there are very few foods which are solely carbohydrates or proteins.

Bread, for instance, contains over 2% protein. So does flour. It is rather difficult to state the amount of protein in cakes, because apart from the protein of the flour, the additional protein depends on the number of eggs added.

A hundred years ago, the food eaten by the working classes in the North of England was 50% bread and potatoes. In those days, workers derived most of their protein from bread, rather than from meat.

Meat and fish are thought of as pure protein foods, but they also contain fat, although they have no carbohydrates in their raw form. But fish in England is mainly eaten fried in a batter containing a large amount of flour. Prepared in this way, fish may contain between 3% to 6% carbohydrates.

The same applies to meat. If it is eaten in the form of stews, casseroles or in pies, a considerable amount of carbohydrates is added to it.

A fashion in some European countries is the 'change-diet' which has been worked out by the two Austrian doctors R. Boller and W. Pilgersdorfer. The slimmers are told to eat proteins combined with carbohydrates for five successive days and then for three days proteins combined with fat, alternately. The diet is easier to follow than the "Hay" diet, but it has also its difficulties. It is not easy to keep strictly to such a diet if one has to take meals away from home.

High Fat Diet

One among nutritionists who recommended this was Pennington in America, in 1953, but some experts point out that a high fat diet had already been used about 100 years earlier by Banting in London. This statement has been repeated so often that today Banting is considered by many to be the originator of the high fat diet.

But was his diet really a high fat diet? Let us find out more about it.

Banting was not a doctor, but a wealthy coffinmaker who at the age of 66 weighed 202 lbs. His height was 5 feet 5 inches. He had tried without success several diets in order to reduce his weight, until in 1862, he consulted an ear, nose and throat surgeon called William Harvey, who put him on a special diet which reduced his weight considerably within several months. He lost 35 lbs. in 38 weeks, and still continued to lose weight until he reached 156 lbs. What was his diet?

Breakfast: Four to five ounces of beef, or mutton, kidneys, boiled fish, bacon or any cold meat except pork. A large cup of tea without sugar or milk and a small biscuit or one ounce of dry toast.

Dinner: Five to six ounces of meat, except pork, or fish, except salmon. Any kind of poultry or game. Any vegetable except potatoes. One ounce of dry toast, some fruit and two to three glasses of good claret, sherry or madeira.

Tea: Two to three ounces of fruit. A rusk or two, and a cup of tea without sugar or milk.

Supper: Three to four ounces of meat or fish, and a glass or two of claret.

For a nightcap he took a tumbler of grog without sugar, or a glass or two of claret or sherry.

Is this really a high fat diet? We notice that he avoided pork when eating meat, and salmon when eating fish. Pork and salmon are well known for their high fat content. We also find that he ate dry toast or rusk. Had he considered fat a harmless food, he would have added butter to the toast or rusk. He drank tea without milk or sugar. Why did he avoid milk? Because milk contains cream among other ingredients.

Some may perhaps say that he also had mutton and

bacon in his diet. Both foods may contain a lot of fat. But as he took particular trouble to avoid fats in other foods, we may safely assume that he chose the lean cuts of mutton and bacon.

From a careful look at his diet, it is obvious that it was a high protein and low carbohydrate diet and not a high fat diet as some people believe. There is nothing miraculous about such a diet. A high protein and low carbohydrate diet has always been advocated for slimming by nutritionists of all schools.

Of course, few would follow such a diet. Eating habits have changed. Not many people today would fancy mutton or beef for breakfast, or grog as a nightcap.

Banting's diet was not even popular in his own time. Few could afford to eat meat three times a day or to drink wine as frequently as Banting did.

In modern times, considerable harm has been done by bizarre fat diets. Foods which contained only traces of carbohydrates were either forbidden to the slimmer or allowed in limited quantities. On the other hand, food with a high fat content was permitted.

I remember one slimming diet given in a newspaper. Slimmers were told to be careful with some vegetables in spite of their low calorie value, but they were allowed to put any amount of butter or margarine on the permitted vegetables.

Which were the "harmful" vegetables? Among others, leeks, carrots and swedes. We must remember that *half a pound* of boiled leeks contains only 56 calories, and the calorie value of carrots and swedes is about the same. All these vegetables are not only harmless but actually suitable for slimmers.

Even well-trained dieticians have been influenced by the avalanche of these articles. I remember a very stout girl of fourteen whom I saw in a school clinic. She complained of pain in her feet, mainly after long standing or walking. An examination of her feet showed no abnormality; the pain was caused by the great weight which she had to carry. When I advised her to reduce her weight, the girl told me that she was receiving treatment from a dietician at a local hospital. I was told that among various foods which she was not allowed to eat were carrots. But she was permitted to eat any amount of cheese. Unfortunately, carrots were the only low calorie vegetable she liked. As she had to dispense with them, she ate cheese instead (two ounces after lunch and supper). By so doing she added at least 350 calories to her food intake. But this was not all. During my questioning, it also became obvious that she did not adhere strictly to all the regulations of her new diet. She continued to eat the same quantity of bread as before. As she was now permitted to eat a liberal amount of butter, she added more butter to the bread than previously. Needless to say that the girl did not reduce her weight. When I saw her several months later, her weight had increased.

The lengths some people went to, to find even minute quantities of carbohydrates in foods and then to warn slimmers to avoid them may be seen from an article which appeared in 1963 in an American medical journal. Here the authors advised dieters to avoid all nuts except the English walnut because it contained smaller amounts of carbohydrate than other nuts.

If people could strictly adhere to diets which forbid the intake of even small quantities of carbohydrates, they would, of course, soon lose all their overweight. But this is impossible, because most foods do contain carbohydrates.

It is, of course, true to say that a high fat diet, so rightly observed by the British nutritionist John Yudkin, was in fact a low calorie diet. We cannot eat a lot of fat if we are not allowed to combine it with carbohydrates. We cannot eat butter or margarine on its own. We smear them on bread or mix them with other carbohydrate-foods, such as flour, in cakes, etc. But fat diets forbid carbohydrates.

We are told, of course, that in such diets we may put any amount of margarine and butter on some of the permitted green vegetables, such as cabbage, brussels sprouts, etc. But, in Britain low calorie vegetables are eaten without any additions (an excellent eating habit!). Only some of the potato dishes, such as roast potatoes, chips or creamed potatoes are made with butter or margarine. But potatoes are forbidden in a fat diet because of their content of carbohydrates. This really means to say that butter or margarine cannot be eaten in large quantities. Thus we save a great amount of calories.

Many estimates have been made of the amount of calories which Banting was supposed to have consumed daily when he was dieting. I have seen books where the authors estimated Banting's daily calorie intake as low as 1,600 and others where his intake was considered to have been as high as 2,800 calories. It is, of course, impossible to give today an accurate estimate of his daily calorie intake. But it cannot have been as high as some writers think, otherwise he would not have lost so much weight in such a short time.

Since high fat diets have been publicised some people have tried to convince overweight people how easy it is to follow them. As an example, slimmers have been told that Eskimos live on high fat diets without feelings of distaste. But we are not Eskimos fortunately. So their delicacies would be repugnant to us, even if we prepared them our own way. How many of us would be able to get used to blubber, walrus—or sealmeat?

Post-war experience has shown that the British could

not even get used to lean whale meat, although it was prepared in the same way as any other meat.

Neither would any of us fancy such ice-cream as Eskimos eat. It consists of crushed ice and raw fat.

Remember that an Eskimo's energy expenditure is very high compared with ours. An Eskimo has to ski or walk beside the dog-drawn sledge for many hours. He has to build igloos or go out hunting under arctic conditions. Some nutritionists estimate his calorie requirements at between 5,000 and 6,000 per day. Nor has an Eskimo the opportunity to eat his meals three times a day as we do. He may go sometimes for a considerable period without food. The eating of fat is a necessity for him, because fat makes him full, and remains longest in the stomach. He therefore does not become hungry so quickly.

The extent to which an Eskimo can fill his stomach may appear unbelievable to many of us, but here is an interesting report which the arctic explorer Lyon made in his Private Journal in 1824. He invited an Eskimo for lunch and noticed what he ate at this one meal.

Of the solid foods the Eskimo consumed:

Breaddust and train oil	1 lb.	10 oz.
Walrus flesh, boiled	7 lb.	1 oz.
Seal and bread	1 lb.	0 oz.
Two candles		3 oz.
Bread and butter		1 oz.
Together he ate	9 lb.	15 oz.

The fluids which the Eskimo consumed at the same meal were:

Rich walrus soup	2 quarts
Water	4 quarts
Together he consumed	6 quarts

Even a glutton in this country would not be able to eat half this amount of food at a single meal, even if it were Westernised food.

This is a report which goes back over 150 years. We have changed since then, Eskimos probably also eat differently now. Nevertheless, they are probably still capable of eating quantities of food at one meal which would be impossible for us.

Saturated and Unsaturated Fats

A final word about the controversies which have arisen during the past decades about the possible dangers of some fats.

It was observed a long time ago that diseases of the heart and of the blood vessels were more common among obese than among lean people. An increased amount of cholesterol was often present in the blood of people suffering from these diseases. Several eminent nutritionists have blamed the increased intake of saturated fats (animal fats), such as lard, butter, cream from milk, meat fat, for the increased cholesterol content in the blood.

It has also been found that some unsaturated fats (mainly vegetable and fish oils) such as corn oil, cottonseed oil, safflower oil, fish oils, lowered the amount of cholesterol in the blood. People having high blood cholesterol levels were therefore advised to omit animal fats and eggs from their diets (the yolk of an egg contains a high amount of cholesterol), and to eat instead some of the vegetable and fish oils.

But a number of nutritionists of equally high reputation have considered the high consumption of carbohydrates, mainly sugar, as the cause of the increase in cholesterol in the blood. Our body can produce cholesterol internally. A high calorie intake may also raise the amount of blood cholesterol. We know that the consumption of sugar in this country has increased enormously. Some nutritionists blame sugar entirely for the cause of obesity and of high blood cholesterol levels.

Whatever the final outcome of this controversy, it is still advisable to cut down on any high calorie foods and reduce one's body weight. Lean people rarely have high blood cholesterol levels.

Incidentally, some doctors, who adhere to the theory that animal fats are the cause of increased blood cholesterol, advise patients suffering from this condition to use vegetable margarines. But this is an error. By converting vegetable oils into margarine (this is done by the action of hydrogen in the presence of a nickel catalyst) the unsaturated fatty acids of the oils are turned into saturated fatty acids. Margarine becomes a saturated fat like animal fat. It is therefore incorrect to include even vegetable margarine among the unsaturated fats.

Eat Less

Some people advise you to continue eating your customary foods, but just eat less of everything. This appears to exempt the slimmer from many difficulties. It sounds quite feasible and understandable. If a person's intake has been about 3,000 calories per day and he then halves all his food portions, he reduces his calorie intake by half. With a diet of 1,500 calories per day he is bound to lose weight, no matter what type of food he is eating.

But from my own experience I know now the danger of this. I learned the hard way. In the beginning everything seemed to go all right although I was always hungry because I was not used to eating small helpings of foods. Nevertheless I lost weight steadily. Within nine months I had shed all my overweight. Eventually my weight came to a standstill although I continued eating the same food portions as I had done while actively slimming. This was to be expected. After having lost so much weight, my energy expenditure had also decreased and I now needed fewer calories to retain my weight.

But I was always hungry because I had not learned proper eating habits. I had to carry on eating small food portions in order not to gain weight. The consequences were disastrous. Six months after having lost all my overweight, I began to suffer from a duodenal ulcer. When I had an X-ray examination I found out how wrong had been the slimming method I had followed. The radiologist informed me that I had a quick emptying stomach. By eating small quantities of foods, my stomach and duodenum were soon empty, and the walls of these two organs were almost continuously exposed to the action of the digestive juices. It was not surprising that an ulcer was the final result.

It took three years for the ulcer to heal. But a year after my ulcer had started I had regained my previous weight because the ulcer diet consisted of high calorie foods which had to be eaten at regular and frequent intervals.

The danger of getting an ulcer after following some slimming methods are hardly ever mentioned by experts although it has long been known that ulcers rarely occur in people who overeat, but far more frequently in people who eat little and keep their stomachs empty for long hours.

Curiously enough, stomach and duodenal ulcers also rarely occur in people who have been exposed to long spells of fasting. It is most probable that by depriving the body completely of food one also stops or greatly diminishes the production of gastric juice.

Eat Slowly

Slimmers are always being advised to eat slowly. The

UNSOUND AND INEFFECTIVE SLIMMING METHODS

reason is logical. The slower we eat, the less food we need. But can we eat as slowly as all that? Fat people are often fast eaters and slim people generally eat rather slowly. Watch this in restaurants. Some diners may still be at the first course, when others at a neighbouring table have finished the third course, even though they had started at the same time.

I have always suspected that slim people who are such slow eaters are so not because of good eating habits, but because they lack a normal appetite. You can observe this better in children. Have you ever watched a child eating a dish he does not like? Did you notice how long it took him to finish it, if he ever did? Enough to bring his mother to despair. But give the child a dish he likes (which is usually sweet), and he soon eats it up.

Adults who are noticeably slow eaters do not seem to have any favourite dishes. They appear to suffer from a general lack of appetite. Whatever foods they are given, they do not seem to enjoy them. It takes them ages to finish a single course. They even leave some of the food on the plate. Somehow, they never seem to be hungry.

Slow eating is not easy for some people. The sense of taste and smell tires very quickly. To enjoy the taste of food, one has to eat it rather quickly. Food which is chewed too long in the mouth loses its savour. Try it with an apple.

In the early years of this century the food fad Horace Fletcher preached a most peculiar method of slow eating. He advised people to chew each morsel of food at least thirty times before swallowing it. He even suggested that they should not swallow milk immediately, but that they "chew" it in the same way.

A piece of chicken must have tasted like blotting paper after being chewed thirty times.

Some of the starchy foods change their taste completely when they are chewed for a long time. They acquire a sweetish taste. Try for instance to chew a piece of fresh, crisp bread the "Fletcher" way. You will notice that the bread gradually acquires an insipid sweet taste. This is because the enzyme Ptyalin, which is in the saliva, has broken down the starch to maltose, which has a sweet taste. When we eat bread at a normal rate, we never experience this because the digestion of starch is a slow process which starts in the mouth, is continued in the stomach and finished in the small intestines.

What has been said so far does not mean that we have to bolt down food in order to enjoy it. Quite the reverse. Many disorders of the stomach can be caused by food which is not properly masticated.

The Effect of Activity in Weight Reducing

This is a divisive controversy.

Some people do not rate exercise very highly as an aid to slimming and consider the omission of a slice of bread to be more important than a long walk. Others have calculated that a daily walk of one mile must lead to a loss of 12 lbs. in weight per year. We have already seen the error of such calculations in Chapter 3.

There is no doubt that activity helps to prevent obesity. Workers who are active throughout their working hours, and who often engage in other physical activities in their free time, will rarely become fat, unless they eat excessively. It is people in sedentary occupations and who also spend their leisure hours in reading and watching television, who are more prone to become overweight. Fortunately, however, there are still sedentary workers who remain slim thanks to other activities and sensible eating habits.

It is not surprising that the incidence of obesity has

UNSOUND AND INEFFECTIVE SLIMMING METHODS

steadily increased. Gone are the days when work at home and outside required great energy expenditure. Today, most housewives no longer have to cope with the heavy tasks which were common fifty years ago.

Thanks to the spread of various labour-saving appliances and machines, of new and easily-cleaned fabrics and coverings, the drudgery has been taken out of household work, so affording the housewife new found leisure.

Similarly, in industry and agriculture, machines now perform much more quickly and efficiently many of the processes that were done slowly by hand or with simple tools.

The number of working hours has also been cut down.

This does not mean that industrial or agricultural workers produce less today than did their predecessors fifty years ago. With the help of modern machines, productivity has greatly increased. Nor does it mean that workers in heavy industries or on the land expend little energy today. They still work very hard. They may still expend 1,000 to 2,000 calories more than people in sedentary jobs.

People in sedentary occupations expend little energy at work, no matter how great may be their mental strain or responsibility. Brain work, unfortunately, is of little significance calorie-wise.

The important question: "Of what value is activity in weight reduction?" is, therefore, not easy to answer. Activity has different effects on different people and may vary from a few short exercises to long hours of energy expenditure at work.

Irregular and short exercises during free time are no substitute for the long and steady activities of miners, steelworkers, etc. A few games of tennis, a few hours of exercise in reducing salons or in the garden cannot greatly reduce the weight of an overweight person if he does not change his eating habits. Sensible eating is the first requirement.

The fatter a person the less strenuous should be his exercise. The heart of a fat person is exposed to great strain which increases with his overweight. Especially after the age of forty, strenuous exercises can be dangerous for very fat people. Even in young overweight people the heart has a hard task to perform. Very fat children and adolescents are soon puffing and panting for breath if they are exposed to strenuous physical activities. No wonder that fat youngsters dislike games!

Very fat people should at first pay more attention to diet than to exercise. Later, when they have lost a considerable amount of fat and the heart is no longer working as hard, they may resume some of the heavier exercises.

This, of course, does not mean that even very fat people should exclude themselves completely from any physical activity. They need light exercises such as gentle walks. Complete inactivity is just as dangerous to them as overstrain. Attacks of coronary thrombosis which are so common in fat people are due not only to overweight but also to lack of exercise.

In short, exercise is an important factor in weight reducing, although in certain conditions, such as heavy overweight or sedentary work, more attention should be paid to diet than to physical activity.

15
Difficulties in Slimming

LONG-ESTABLISHED eating habits cannot be effortlessly abandoned. It is difficult to give up some of the low calorie accessory foods to which one has long been accustomed. An Englishman sorely misses his cup of tea and a Frenchman, an Italian or a Spaniard his customary glass of wine with his meals.

It is worse still for a person suddenly to be reduced to a very low calorie diet if he has been accustomed to richer meals.

Expense

It is easy to tell people to go on high protein diets, but it is not so easy to follow them. High protein diets are very expensive. It is senseless to tell a poorly paid person, whose work prevents him from dining at home, to eat large portions of steak in restaurants. Even at home, lean beef is probably beyond his means.

Religious Scruples

Nor is it possible for people of certain religions to follow diets which are forbidden to them. An orthodox Jew or Moslem will not eat pork, nor a Hindu, beef.

Personal and National Aversions

A person may have such an aversion to certain foods that it is useless to instruct him to eat them. Dislikes for some foods may even be a national characteristic. The Japanese, for instance, are nauseated at the sight of butter and certain other fats.

Some people are convinced that certain foods "disagree" with them or cause them indigestion, even though there is no justification for this assumption. It would be hopeless for the doctor to try to persuade them to the contrary. I knew a man who could not be persuaded to eat cabbage or tomatoes because he was convinced that they caused him indigestion, but he ate pickled cucumbers with relish. I also remember a patient who found apples to be indigestible, but he liked eating oranges which act no differently from apples on the stomach and bowels.

Allergies

In some cases a person's sensitivity to some foods can be so great as to result in a severe skin rash. The skin of some people, especially children, may react strongly to eggs, shellfish, strawberries, tomatoes, parsnips and several other foods. It is therefore futile for these foods to be prescribed to them.

Lack of Variety of Diets

A complaint often made by slimmers is the monotony and tastelessness of slimming diets. This difficulty could be alleviated if people were more familiar with calorie values. They would then be able to choose from a greater variety of low calorie foods and not be limited to the few food items mentioned in their diet sheets.

Constipation

Some people complain of constipation while slimming. This condition could also be easily remedied if slimmers would learn more about calorie values. Low calorie vegetables and fresh fruits are very effective on constipation.

The Dieter who is "Odd Man Out"

Some slimmers, especially housewives, find it tantalizing to abstain from their high calorie favourite foods whilst watching other members of the family eat them. This difficulty would disappear if only they knew more about the astronomic calorie levels of some of their favourite dishes. They would then be less tempted to eat them. I have to face the same difficulty when having my daily lunch in restaurants and watching other people. But the knowledge of calories has greatly helped me to surmount this obstacle.

Relatives and Friends

A difficulty which most slimmers have to face is the unhelpful attitude of relatives and friends. Like sirens they try to persuade the slimmer to return to his old figure.

"Your new figure does not suit you."
"You will get T.B."
"You are in a state of nervous tension."
"You will soon have a nervous breakdown."
"You should stop dieting for a while."

These are some of the remarks most slimmers have to listen to while dieting. When I had lost only half of my overweight, I even heard the complimentary remark from a friend that it was now time for me to stop dieting because I had lost it all. I could write at length about what I had to listen to during the first stages of slimming. Fortunately, I had an excellent answer for all these sirens: I was then convalescing from a serious illness due to overweight. My friends were nonplussed when I told them that according to the specialist's opinion, only weight reduction could prolong my life.

Though you may have a less valid answer for your

friends and relatives, simply ignore their advice. After all, it is your own health you are concerned about.

Difficulties in Institutions, Restaurants and At Home

While dieting, some slimmers may have special difficulties to face which may vary from person to person. Some may find it difficult to obtain the right food if they live in institutions or boarding houses. Others may find it difficult even in their own homes to prepare the right food for themselves if they have to cater for a large family. My personal difficulty has always been to obtain the right food in restaurants.

I live in a city in the North of England. During my twenty years here I have seen many restaurants open and close down, but I am still waiting for a self-service restaurant which can offer me a one-course meal with two low calorie vegetables.

Among six vegetables which are available in the two largest restaurants, only one is of low calorie value. Here is the selection of vegetables served there: potato chips, creamed potatoes, baked beans, broad beans occasionally, peas, and, on alternate days, cabbage or carrots or turnips. Two low calorie vegetables are never obtainable on the same day. What use is it to advise slimmers to eat plenty of low calorie vegetables if they are not obtainable?

Something else in restaurants is rather puzzling. Why are the portions of low calorie vegetables so small? I live in an agricultural region, well known for its cheap products. But the portions of low calorie vegetables served here in restaurants are minute. Years ago, I once meekly asked the assistant at the service counter of one restaurant to give me a larger helping of cabbage. The look she gave me taught me never again to ask for more vegetable. What would have happened had I asked her to give me another paper-thin slice of roast beef served with the cabbage? Terrible! I dare not think of it.

Only one vegetable is usually obtainable here in large quantities: potato chips. The portions may sometimes be two or three times as large as those of cabbage or carrots.

I suspect that this situation is typical of that throughout Great Britain. It is as if there is a conspiracy to prevent slimmers from getting a square meal.

The only occasion, therefore, when I can feast on low calorie vegetables, salads, meat and fish is when I eat at home. There I often have two or three low calorie vegetables with my meal. The portions of meat and fish I eat at home are far larger than those served in restaurants, and I do not have to count the number of lettuce leaves, tomatoes or slices of cucumber when I eat salad.

Slimmers may often be advised by some writers to avoid restaurants and to take packed lunches to their work. For some, this may be sensible advice, but there are others who are not able to follow it. It is not always easy to get low calorie meals, but the knowledge of calorie values at least teaches us to choose the lesser evil when dining out.

If You are Invited Out for a Meal

A large number of slimmers find social invitations a serious obstacle to their weight reducing regimes. The dishes offered on such occasions are often high in calories. If you are one of those people who have to attend three banquets a week and several more cocktail parties while still wanting to slim, then you might be in trouble. But if, like me, you are invited out to dine about once a month, then take my advice and don't worry. I never diet when I am invited out. I thoroughly enjoy the dinners, I do not even refuse high calorie puddings because I see no harm in occasionally eating a rich meal.

This is why: assuming you consume three meals a day, you then average ninety meals a month. Do you really think that if you diet carefully eighty-nine times during the month, and you eat only one high calorie meal, your weight will rise steeply? This has never happened to me. Since I lost my overweight my weight has always remained constant.

Unfortunately, many people slim just the opposite way. At home or in restaurants they are not very particular about their diet. They will transgress the rules of dieting eighty-nine times a month, but when they are invited out they become shining examples of strict dieters. They often drive a hostess to despair. No food satisfies them. Even a small biscuit is too much. All the hostess hears is: "No, thank you".

Some people do this for years without ever losing an ounce of overweight.

When I mentioned earlier that I did not diet in friends' homes, my statement was not quite correct. I do diet in a small way but it is hardly noticed. I eat very little bread and rarely take more than one sandwich. No hostess will be offended or even notice it if a guest does not empty a plate of bread, but she will be sadly disappointed if he refuses some of her dishes which she has prepared with care.

I remember one evening when I was invited to a friend for dinner. There were other guests there who seemed to belong to the group of "semi-dieters", because they were rather fussy with the food. Our first dish was a fish and egg salad. On the table were also a bread-plate loaded with buttered bread rolls and a bottle of salad cream. None of the guests, except me, touched the salad cream, but they emptied the bread-plate with astonishing rapidity. They did this so quickly that the hostess had to go to the kitchen and prepare a few more rolls. The second round

DIFFICULTIES IN SLIMMING

of rolls soon disappeared too. I had not touched a single roll but my hostess asked me whether I should like some more bread. It was that evening that I realised how little attention is paid to the guests who do not touch bread.

Later, when tea was served, I was the only one who took sugar with the tea. The other guests used saccharine. I was also the only one who accepted a piece of chocolate. A lady sitting next to me was surprised at my "careless" way of eating. She knew that I was on a diet and could not understand how I had dared to eat so many forbidden foods. In fact, she asked me tactfully whether I had given up my diet. Unfortunately, nothing could convince her that *small* quantities of high calorie foods, eaten on *rare* occasions, could not do much harm to the slimmer. But what had she eaten in addition to her meal? I had watched her, too: Two buttered bread rolls which amounted to at least 400 calories. Compared with her I had eaten only very little in excess. The teaspoonful of sugar contained 30 calories, the piece of chocolate hardly more than 50 calories and the two teaspoonfuls of salad cream eaten with the salad amounted to about 60 calories. In all, I had consumed about 140 calories, still only a fraction of the excess 400 calories which the lady had eaten.

Later, when sandwiches and cakes were served, I took a thin slice of cake, which could not have contained more than 150 calories. But the same lady who was so surprised at my frequent dietary "transgressions" took two sandwiches which must have amounted to 600 calories. Had she only known more about the calorie values of some "harmless" foods, she would not have condemned me so much for my "careless" eating.

I do not mean to give the impression that sugar, chocolate and cakes are harmless foods for the slimmer. They are, in fact, the most dangerous foods for him if they are eaten daily and in excess. Neither at home, nor in restaurants or cafeterias do I ever take sugar. Saccharine tablets have become my constant companions for the last twelve years. Nor do I ever eat cakes or chocolates outside a friend's home.

But I never abstain from salad cream at home. One or two teaspoons of salad cream, spread carefully over the greens of a salad may turn insipid rabbit food into a tasty meal, without greatly increasing the calorie content of a salad. The situation is, of course, different if you eat a salad made in the continental style. There, the ingredients of the salad such as pieces of pickled herring, potatoes or other vegetables are literally drenched in enormous quantities of mayonnaise or salad cream. Keep away from such salads. Eat salads prepared the English way.

There may be other difficulties for slimmers. But what he should know is that slimming is not always as easy as some writers claim. Nor is it as difficult as others imagine. A better knowledge of calorie values will help the slimmer to make the right decisions.

16
The Slimming Secret

WHAT *is* the right way to slim? What can be done to lose superfluous weight safely and permanently?

It would be impossible to work out a standard diet which would suit every slimmer. Your weight reducing diet may be completely different from that of others because your energy expenditures may differ. It would be illogical to suggest a slimming diet which would equally well suit a miner, a woman of seventy, a child of ten or an adolescent of eighteen, if all four are overweight. Unfortunately, standard diets which are supposed to fit every slimmer are still being published. These attempts show a high failure rate.

Learn the Calorie Values of Foods

As an individual you have to find out your own diet. It is not easy to do this, but less hard than you may imagine. Your first step is to become acquainted with calorie values. Once you know them, you will be able to differentiate high-calorie from low-calorie foods, and you must learn to avoid foods of a high calorie content. You will also learn why you have become overweight and you will realise that some of the foods, which you have been eating so carelessly, were not of such low calorie value as you thought.

Lose Weight Slowly

The next step is to try to lose your weight slowly. I

repeat: *slowly*! It is useless to shed your overweight quickly by some bizarre crash diets and then to resume your old eating habits. By so doing, your old weight is bound to come back again. The more slowly you slim the more likely you are to lose your overweight permanently. Why? Because new eating habits can only be formed gradually if you want to adhere to them for the rest of your life. This has been my own experience. It took me a full year to lose my overweight of 40 lbs. But this slow method had its rewards. I never regained even part of my overweight once I had reached my normal weight and I have retained this weight for the last eleven years.

Shun Intolerable Diets

Losing weight is not like an appendix operation. Once an appendix has been removed by an operation it never grows again. But lost weight is bound to return if correct eating habits are not practised throughout life.

Next time you hear of a miracle cure, promising you a great loss of weight within a short time, ask yourself: "Can I maintain this diet for the rest of my life?" If not, keep away from it. You will only experience frustration within a short time of finishing the cure. Your lost weight will return with amazing speed, because you have not learned permanent good eating habits.

Changes in Eating Habits should be Gentle and Gradual

What then is the better and easier method of losing weight permanently? Instead of drastically changing all your bad eating habits overnight, try at first to avoid one or two of your usual high calorie foods. But please, not more than one or two in the beginning. If you are used, for instance, to eating pudding with one of your meals and to having tea or coffee with sugar, omit the pudding or replace it by fresh fruit, and substitute saccharine for sugar. It is not difficult to begin with one or two changes in your diet. Later, when your weight loss comes to a standstill, and you still need further weight reduction, you will have to cut down on some other high calorie foods and replace them by foods of lower calorie content. This was the slimming method which I used when I finally succeeded, and I lost 20 lbs. during my first six months of slimming.

The Hidden Dangers of Drastic Changes

Why did I use this slow method? When I left hospital after a very serious illness caused by obesity, it became essential for me to lose my overweight. I was then 40 lbs. overweight, and I had to lose it to have any chance of survival. I studied a number of diets which promised a quick loss of weight only to realise that I was not suitable for such methods.

Most of these diets allowed only three meals per day. The permitted foods were not only low in calories but were also small in quantity. Besides, many of these diets forbade the intake of food—not even tea or coffee—between meals. I had already suffered from a duodenal ulcer which was caused by eating small quantities of food and by abstention from food between meals. I knew that by following such a diet my old ulcer would soon flare up again.

Fortunately, I had already gained some insight into the calorie values of foods, and I decided to cut out, at first, only one or two of the high calorie foods and to await the results. The omission of pudding replaced by an apple and the substitution of saccharine for sugar in tea and coffee became my first step. To my pleasant surprise, these two changes alone caused a gradual drop in my weight. In terms of calories this was quite understandable.

The daily omission of a helping of pudding weighing four ounces amounted to a loss of 400 calories. Although I replaced the pudding by an apple (50 calories) the loss was still 350 calories. The six teaspoonfuls of sugar which I replaced by saccharine in my daily tea and coffee meant a saving of another 180 calories. Thus, I saved 530 calories per day or 3,710 calories per week, quite a substantial reduction seeing that I had made only two changes in my daily eating habits. Six months later I was 20 lbs. lighter.

The Plateau in Weight Reduction

Then my weight became stationary in spite of the continued omission of pudding and sugar. During the next four weeks I neither lost nor gained weight. It was obvious that a standstill which some nutritionists call the plateau of weight reduction, had occurred. After losing 20 lbs., my body no longer carried as much weight as before, so my energy expenditure had decreased and so did my food requirements. But, as I was still 20 lbs. overweight, I needed to reduce still further my food intake in order to lose my remaining overweight.

Watch your Intake of Bread

By now I had become well acquainted with calorie values and realised that, apart from pudding and sugar, my large consumption of bread had also been a source of my high calorie intake. Since childhood I had always been a great bread eater. This bad eating habit originated during the years immediately after the First World War when food was very scarce and it remained with me in later years when food was no longer rationed. I continued to eat bread with most courses of my meals. To me it had become just as important as salt. Meals would have tasted insipid without it.

When, however, I became acquainted with calorie values I realised how many calories I had been consuming with my daily bread intake. This dangerous habit had to be stopped, but not suddenly, because it had been established far too long.

Gradually I began to omit bread with some meals. First I learned to eat meat and vegetables without bread. This was not an easy task but somehow I succeeded. It may perhaps seem odd that to give up bread with this course of the meal demanded so much effort because it is not customary to eat bread with meat and vegetables. But for me it was quite a difficult task. Later I gave up eating bread and butter or sandwiches between meals, taking instead either fruit, tea or coffee. Finally, I cut down on bread at breakfast and replaced most of it with fruit.

It is difficult to give up old established eating habits suddenly. Some people find it impossible. But I learned that it *is* possible to give up old eating habits if one does so very slowly and gradually. Years ago I would have found it impossible to eat fruit for breakfast. But in time I got used to eating an apple with a slice of bread and butter for breakfast, and I do not find anything odd about this practice now.

Substituting Low Calorie Foods for High Ones

Having lost my superfluous 40 lbs., I soon learned that a further reduction in my daily calorie intake had to be made, in order to keep my new weight steady. This was because my energy expenditure had dropped considerably by now. Here again the knowledge of the calorie value of foods came as a great help to me.

Gradually I learned to substitute other low calorie foods. Potato chips were the next item to disappear from my meals. They were replaced gradually by boiled potatoes or potatoes baked in their jackets. It was a slow process, so that today I cannot say when I finally stopped eating chips. I only know now that I have not eaten them for a number of years. Fried fish and fat meat were other foods which gradually vanished from my meals. They were replaced by grilled fish and lean meat.

It would, of course, be wrong to advise every slimmer to follow my personal pattern of weight reducing. Some may not be eating puddings or taking sugar with tea or coffee. They therefore have to start their slimming regime differently. But they will be able to omit high calorie foods only if they become acquainted with their calorie content and know at what meals they have been consuming their superfluous calories.

Here people vary considerably. Some, for instance, eat most of their high calorie foods during their main meals. There are many calories hidden in creamed soups (which are also often eaten with bread), in fried fish, in meat pies, meat puddings, sausages, spaghetti, noodles, macaroni, dumplings, fried potatoes, fried rice, baked beans, gravies, puddings, etc., and also in cheese which is so often eaten as the last course of a main meal. The omission of one or two of these regularly eaten high calorie foods would make a good start in slimming. Later, of course, slimmers would have to cut down more.

Watch Your Accessory Foods

There are others who do not derive their superfluous calories from main meals but from food eaten between meals. Sandwiches, biscuits, doughnuts, cakes, pastries, chocolate, tea or coffee sweetened with sugar are often taken between meals and may add considerably to the daily calorie intake.

In some homes (and institutions) there still exists the custom of a rich 4 o'clock tea. I dare not think of the opulent 4 o'clock teas which I used to take for several years when I worked in hospitals. They often exceeded the calories of some of the main meals. We used to have sandwiches, cakes, buttered bread, scones, jam, tea and sugar, and we could eat as much as we liked.

Is It Always Wise to Abstain From Food Between Meals?

Many writers on slimming forbid eating or drinking between meals. This is not always sound. It may cause a great strain and severe hunger pangs. If a person takes a low calorie mid-day meal at 12 o'clock and then has to wait six or seven hours for his evening meal without even a drink, he will arrive home ravenous. He will then probably be unable to control his food intake. In such a situation the mind no longer has the power to rule over a very hungry stomach.

Many slimming experts seem to ignore this fact. They even state that small meals cause the stomach to shrink within a short time, so that even with small food portions you feel full for longer intervals. This never happened to me.

Complete abstention from foods between meals is certainly not the right way to slim, unless you are one of the exceptional few who can really manage to go without for a considerable time without finding it an ordeal.

I always take between meals a cup of tea or coffee which is served where I work. In addition, I often take tea in cafés or at home about half an hour before my main meals. This practice has saved me from sitting down hungry at my main meals, and, consequently, from eating more than necessary.

It is most important that you should never start a meal feeling very hungry. If you do, you may be unable to limit yourself to small helpings. A hungry stomach always requires larger quantities of food. When you begin to feel hungry before a meal, take a cup of tea, but not one sweetened with sugar. The drink will fill and pacify your growling stomach for a short while and will take the edge off your appetite.

Some people may perhaps think it odd to take a hot drink shortly before a meal, as it is customary in England to drink tea or coffee *after* a meal. Some will even say that drinking tea or coffee before meals spoils the appetite. But is this not just what a slimmer needs?

The Danger of Unconscious Eating

There exists a type of person who eats sensibly during the day, but who consumes excess calories during the evening hours. This phenomenon has long been known by nutritionists and is called the *night eating syndrome*. Such people may eat large amounts of foods without even being conscious of doing so. How many people are aware of the many titbits they consume whilst watching television programmes?

Unconscious overeating need not be confined to the evening hours. There are men who can ingest a considerably number of slices of toast or buttered bread at breakfast, while they are deeply absorbed in a newspaper. If you ask them afterwards how many slices they have eaten, they have no idea. The same happens with youngsters when they are engrossed in comics or adventure books. They may eat enormous quantities of sweets without being aware of it.

What is the cure for such unconscious eating? Answer, knowledge of calorie values. Once you know them, you will not overeat so lightheartedly. Years ago I would not have known how much bread I had eaten during a day; today I can account for every slice.

Examples of Excessive Calorie Intake

There are people who derive their extra calories in a rather unusual way. Remember, for example, the bus driver who gained so much weight merely from drinking numerous cups of tea and coffee sweetened with plenty of sugar.

People also gain a lot of weight solely by drinking excessive amounts of beer. One of them told me that he drank eight to ten pints of beer every evening.

One case I remember was a boy of twelve with a colossal weight, whom I saw many years ago. From his mother I heard a rather sad story. At home the boy had always been brought up with sensible eating habits. But he had indulgent grandparents who daily gave him a lot of pocket money, enough to buy a pound of cheap sweets daily. With these he must have added at least 1,500 calories daily to his ordinary food intake. 10,500 calories per week! Had the grandparents given him a pound of fresh fruit instead of the money, he would have consumed only 200 extra calories daily. Per week he would have consumed about 9,000(!) calories fewer than with sweets. Had his grandparents had some insight into calorie values they could have saved the boy from his excessive weight.

How and When to Weigh Yourself

If you want to know how effective your weight reduction programme is you have to weigh yourself weekly, not only while you are losing weight, but also after you have reached your normal weight. Weighing should become your lifelong habit.

At first, do not weigh yourself more than once a week. Do not expect to see results within a few days. Even on a very drastic diet you won't see immediate results.

Once you have noticed a loss in weight, continue to weigh yourself weekly, preferably on the same scale, and at the same time of day (the best time is after breakfast). If you have no scale at home, and you weigh yourself outside, allow for the fact that the weight of your clothes varies from season to season. If you slip up occasionally with your diet it may not be pleasant to go on a scale afterwards, but you must steel yourself to do this if you seriously want to look after your weight.

The mistake so often made by slimmers is to weigh themselves frequently while weight is being lost, but to stop after the normal weight has been reached.

Why Some Slimmers Do Not Lose Weight Immediately

Some people do not lose weight during their first few weeks of slimming, no matter how strict their diet. But this apparent failure to lose weight should not discourage them, because they really do lose fat. However, their weight remains constant in the beginning because their body tends to retain a considerable amount of water during the first weeks of weight reduction. Why this should happen with some people but not with others has never been discovered.

Some women tend to retain a lot of water during their periods so that they show increased weight at such times.

These facts need not necessarily apply to you. You may perhaps experience a drop in weight within a week or two after the start of your slimming. But if you belong to that group of people whose weight remains constant during the first few weeks (this period may even last as long as a month) do not despair. Provided you can earnestly say that you have been omitting 500 calories daily from your usual food intake, you should in time be able to see good results.

Why It Is Essential to Know Your Calories

The reason I have put so much emphasis on the knowledge of calorie values is that I have found it *the most important guide* for slimmers. Understanding calories has not only freed me from my persistent overweight throughout many years, but has also prevented me from regaining my previous weight. The knowledge of calories has also taught me that occasional transgressions in dieting are not too detrimental to a slimmer at times when it is impossible to adhere to the strict rules.

If you are scared of occasional rich meals, knowledge of calories will teach you to cut down on some of your daily foods a few days before a special event. You can then enjoy large dinners with a clear conscience.

There are other occasions during the year which you cannot avoid, especially if you have a family which enjoys them. For instance, are you going to deny yourself a holiday because you are afraid that the meals served away from home will not conform to your daily diet? In most European countries eating habits are different from those in Great Britain. There you won't be served with bacon and eggs in the morning. Bread rolls, butter, jam and coffee are more usual. And so with other meals abroad. But if you are familiar with calories, you will know which of the foreign foods to eat sparingly and which to enjoy freely. You will even find abroad quite a few savoury foods of low calorie content which you will later copy frequently at home. I often eat low calorie dishes which I discovered years ago while holidaying abroad.

If you gain a few pounds in weight while on holiday you need not worry unduly. They will always disappear once you resume ordinary eating habits.

Many nutritionists rightly point out that apart from knowledge of calorie values, the recognition of the composition of foods is equally important to the slimmer. Foods such as proteins and carbohydrates may be equal in calorie value, but they may be of different importance to the slimmer. The slimmer should always take proteins in preference to carbohydrates, yet carbohydrates need not be completely discarded from a slimming cure. Vegetables or fruits may also be equal in calorie value to smaller quantities of other foods such as chocolate, but the former should always be eaten in preference to the latter.

In many circumstances advice like this should not be necessary. Common sense will tell the slimmer what to choose. A two ounce bar of chocolate, for instance, contains just over 300 calories. On the other hand two ounces of lean roast beef with a boiled potato and a good helping of cauliflower also contains about 300 calories. Surely every slimmer knows instinctively which of these to choose for a main meal?

This last example may be rather too obvious. Other choices could cause the slimmer greater difficulty. To spare him this, I have marked in the calorie tables symbols which will help him to choose the right foods. They show which foods are dangerous for the slimmer, which he should avoid if possible, which he may eat in moderation or as normal helpings, and which he may eat in any quantity he likes.

Even these symbols should not be taken too narrowly. Alcohol, for instance, drunk regularly, is certainly a menace to the slimmer so that alcoholic beverages are marked in the calorie table as dangerous. But a glass of beer, or a small glass of wine or spirits, taken occasionally at some social event is not going to cause much harm.

This principle applies to other foods of high calorie value, which are marked in the table as dangerous, but which can be eaten quite frequently in very small quantities combined with large quantities of low calorie foods.

Salad cream, for instance, in small amounts is probably a "must" for your salads. It has certainly not increased my weight, and it will not harm you either.

Many other examples could be given. I know a lady who is an expert in making delicious clear chicken soups of very low calorie value. One day she confided to me the secret of her tasty soup. She added a teaspoonful of sugar to the soup made for about six people. But she asked me not to disclose the secret to her other guests because they would not eat it if they knew that there was sugar in it. It sounds incredible that people should refuse such a tiny amount of sugar. A teaspoonful of sugar contains 30 calories. Added to a soup for six people it means a negligible 5 calories per person. But many people think that this insignificant amount of sugar will cause a great increase in their weight. Ironically enough, these same people would not hesitate to eat bread with the soup, although bread contains a great amount of carbohydrate, and may have twenty times as many calories as this small quantity of sugar.

Are Eggs Safe for the Slimmer?

There are several nutritional problems which have not yet been entirely solved, so that they have made the precise marking of the calorie tables difficult. For instance, a controversy still rages about whether eggs are safe for all slimmers. Eggs contain protein of a high quality and they are low in calories, properties ideal for the slimmer. But the yolk of an egg contains a high amount of cholesterol which may be dangerous for those who have had a thrombosis of a heart or brain vessel, or are suffering from hardening of the arteries. Some nutritionists do not consider eggs to be dangerous for such conditions, others restrict sufferers to one egg a week.

Although I have marked eggs in the enclosed calorie

table as suitable foods for slimmers, they should be eaten by the young rather than by elderly people.

My Hope for the Slimmer

I hope that this book has shown overweight people some of the wrong ways they have followed, and that it has freed them from erroneous beliefs about slimming.

Now they may realise that they are not unhappy martyrs who have been destined by fate to remain fat, no matter how little they eat. I hope that those who have been unsuccessful with slimming diets have now found a more rational way of losing overweight and that they will achieve a permanent normal weight.

CALORIE GUIDE FOR THE OVERWEIGHT

Key to the Symbols

- ●●● Danger—be careful.
- ●● Avoid it—if possible.
- ● Eat it in moderation.
- ★ Eat normal helpings.
- ★★ Eat any amount you like.

BREADS

"The poet's fate is here in emblem shown, he asked for bread and he gained a stone."
  (With apologies to Samuel Wesley.)

	Calories in 4 oz.	Normal Helping	Calories in Normal Helping
Bread, brown	●● 272	1 slice, 1 oz.	68
Bread, hovis	●● 268	1 slice, 1 oz.	67
Bread, malt	●● 284	1 slice, 1 oz.	71
Bread, white	●● 276	1 slice, 1 oz.	69
Bread, white, fried	●● 648	1 slice, 1 oz.	162
Bread, white, toasted	●● 340	1 slice, 1 oz.	85
Bread crumbs, white	●● 404	1 oz.	101
Energen rolls	● 444	1 roll	18
Figger rolls	● 440	1 roll	18
Holland rusk	●● 420	1 rusk, $\frac{2}{3}$ oz.	70
Rye bread (continental)	●● 312	1 slice, 1 oz.	75
Ryvita	● 392	1 piece	25
Vienna bread	●● 304	1 slice, 1 oz.	76

SANDWICHES

Plain sandwich: *260 calories* ●●
Two slices of bread (1 oz. each): 140 calories
Two pats of butter (or margarine): 120 calories

Toast sandwich (plain): *290 calories* ●●
Two slices of toast (1 oz. each): 170 calories
Two pats of butter (or margarine): 120 calories

Breakfast toast, one slice (with marmalade and butter):
 185 calories ●●

One slice of toast: 85 calories
One pat of butter (or margarine): 60 calories
½ oz. marmalade: 40 calories

Cheese sandwich: *380 calories* ●●
Two slices of bread (1 oz. each): 140 calories
Two pats of butter (or margarine): 120 calories
1 oz. of cheese (Cheshire): 120 calories

Corned beef sandwich: *326 calories* ●●
Two slices of bread: 140 calories
Two pats of butter (or margarine): 120 calories
1 oz. of corned beef: 66 calories

Egg and tomato sandwich: *305 calories* ●●
Two slices of bread: 140 calories
Two pats of butter (or margarine): 120 calories
Half an egg: 35 calories
One tomato: 10 calories

Ham sandwich: *380 calories* ●●
Two slices of bread: 140 calories
Two pats of butter (or margarine): 120 calories
1 oz. of ham: 120 calories

THE SLIMMING SECRET

Salmon sandwich: *300 calories*
Two slices of bread: 140 calories
Two pats of butter (or margarine): 120 calories ●●
1 oz. of salmon: 40 calories

CEREALS

*"Needles and pins, needles and pins,
A breakfast with cereals, and trouble begins."*
(Variation on an old nursery rhyme.)

	Calories in 4 oz.	Normal Helping	Calories in Normal Helping
All Bran	●● 352	1 oz.	88
Barley pearl, raw	●● 408	1 oz.	102
Barley pearl, boiled	●● 136	3 oz.	102
Cornflakes	●● 416	1 oz.	104
Cornflour	●● 400	½ oz.	50
Flour	●● 400	½ oz.	50
Grapenuts	●● 408	1 oz.	102
Macaroni, raw	●● 408	2 oz.	204
Macaroni, boiled	●● 128	6 oz.	192
Oatmeal, raw	●● 460	1 oz.	115
Oatmeal, porridge	●● 52	8 oz.	104
Puffed-rice	●● 480	1 oz.	120
Rice Krispies	●● 400	1 oz.	100
Rice Flakes	●● 400	1 oz.	100
Rice, raw	●● 408	1 oz.	102
Rice, boiled	●● 140	3 oz.	105
Sago, raw	●● 404	1 oz.	101
Semolina, raw	●● 400	1 oz.	100
Soya flour (whole)	●● 492	1 oz.	123
Soya flour (low fat)	●● 380	1 oz.	95
Spaghetti, raw	●● 416	2 oz.	208
Spaghetti, boiled	●● 136	6 oz.	204
Tapioca	●● 408	1 oz.	102

Wheat:

	Calories in 4 oz.	Normal Helping	Calories in Normal Helping
Flakes	●● 460	1 oz.	115
Krispies	●● 460	1 oz.	115
Puffed	●● 440	1 oz.	110
Shredded	●● 440	1 oz.	110

CAKES, BISCUITS AND PASTRIES

These contain three unsuitable ingredients for the slimmer: flour, sugar, fat. Avoid them like high voltage.

	Calories in 4 oz.	Normal Helping	Calories in Normal Helping
Angel cake	●●● 300	2 oz.	150
Chocolate cake	●●● 564	2 oz.	282
Curd cheese cake	●●● 556	2 oz.	278
Currant bun	●●● 348	2 oz.	174
Devil's food	●●● 450	2 oz.	225
Doughnuts	●●● 404	2 oz.	202
Dundee cake	●●● 440	2 oz.	220
Eccles cake	●●● 588	2 oz.	294
Fruit cake	●●● 428	2 oz.	214
Ginger bread	●●● 432	2 oz.	216
Scones	●●● 420	2 oz.	210
Sponge cake	●●● 348	2 oz.	174

Biscuits: These vary in size and weight. It is therefore impossible to state the exact calorie value of a single biscuit.

Biscuits, Digestive	●●● 548
Biscuits, Ginger	●●● 508
Biscuits, Plain	●●● 492
Biscuits, Sweet	●●● 632
Biscuits, water	●●● 504
Biscuits, Crackers	●●● 632
Biscuits, Shortbread	●●● 592

THE SLIMMING SECRET

	Calories in 4 oz.	Normal Helping	Calories in Normal Helping
Pastries:			
Jam tartlet	●●● 448	1½ oz.	168
Lemon tartlet	●●● 500	1½ oz.	187
Mince pie	●●● 444	2 oz.	222
Custard tartlet	●●● 328	1½ oz.	123
Pies:			
Apple pie	●●● 216	3 oz.	162
Custard pie	●●● 268	3 oz.	201
Gooseberry pie	●●● 204	3 oz.	153
Lemon meringue pie	●●● 268	3 oz.	201
Plum pie	●●● 208	3 oz.	166
Rhubarb pie	●●● 212	3 oz.	159

DAIRY PRODUCTS

These are helpful for slimmers if taken in the right quantities.

	Calories in 4 oz.	Normal Helping	Calories in Normal Helping
Butter:	●● 904	¼ oz.	57
Cheese:			
Blue Danish	● 412	1 oz.	103
Bel Paese	● 360	1 oz.	90
Brie	● 440	1 oz.	110
Camembert	● 352	1 oz.	88
Cheddar	● 480	1 oz.	120
Cheshire	● 440	1 oz.	110
Cottage (from skimmed milk)	★ 128	2 oz.	64
Cream cheese	●● 680	1 oz.	170
Edam	● 352	1 oz.	88
Gouda	● 384	1 oz.	96

	Calories in 4 oz.	Normal Helping	Calories in Normal Helping
Gorgonzola	● 448	1 oz.	112
Grueyére	● 480	1 oz.	120
Limburger	● 300	1 oz.	75
Parmesan	● 480	½ oz. grated	60
Norwegian	● 300	1 oz.	75
Roquefort	● 440	1 oz.	110
Stilton	● 540	1 oz.	135
Wensleydale	● 460	1 oz.	115

Cream:
Heavy	●● 524	1 oz.	131
Light	●● 248	1 oz.	62

Milk:
Whole	● 76	8 oz.	152
Skimmed	★ 40	8 oz.	80
Condensed, sweetened	●● 400	1 oz.	100
Condensed, unsweetened	● 176	1 oz.	44
Evaporated	● 160	½ oz.	20
Malted, dry	●● 420	⅓ oz.	35

Yoghourt	● 160	4 oz.	160

Eggs and egg dishes:
One egg	★		75
Egg white	★		20
Egg yolk	●		55
Egg, boiled	★		75
Egg, fried (+ 1 tsp. fat)	●		130
Egg, poached	★		75
Egg, scrambled (+ tsp. fat + 1 tbsp. milk)	●		150
Omelette (2 eggs):			
Plain	●		200

	Calories in 4 oz.	Normal Helping	Calories in Normal Helping
Omelettes:—			
Cheese (+ ½ oz. Parmesan cheese)	●		260
Jam (+ 1 oz. jam)	●●		270
Mushroom	●		200
Scotch egg	● 300	4 oz.	300

FATS

"Fat flesh freezes soon."
                        (Scottish proverb.)

	Calories in 4 oz.	Normal Helping	Calories in Normal Helping
Beef dripping	●● 1048	½ oz.	131
Butter	●● 904	¼ oz.	57
Cooking fat	●● 1048	½ oz.	131
Lard	●● 1048	½ oz.	131
Margarine	●● 904	½ oz.	113
Mayonnaise	●● 800	½ oz.	100
Olive oil	●● 1056	½ oz.	132
Salad dressing (French)	●● 480	½ oz.	60

FISH AND FISH PRODUCTS

"Fish should swim three times: in water, in sauce and in wine."
                        (French proverb.)

For the slimmer, only in water!

	Calories in 4 oz.	Normal Helping	Calories in Normal Helping
Anchovies	★ 120	½ oz.	15
Bass, raw	● 104	6 oz.	156
Bass, steamed	● 144	4 oz.	144
Bloater	●● 260	4 oz.	260
Bloater paste	● 280	½ oz.	35

	Calories in 4 oz.	Normal Helping	Calories in Normal Helping
Bream, steamed	★ 68	4 oz.	68
Brill, steamed	★ 88	4 oz.	88
Carp, raw	● 160	6 oz.	240
Catfish, steamed	★ 112	4 oz.	112
Clams, raw	★ 92	4 oz.	92
Cockles	★ 56	2 oz.	28
Cod, fried	●● 160	4 oz.	160
steamed	★ 92	4 oz.	92
roe, fried	●● 236	3 oz.	177
Cod liver oil	●● 1040	½ oz.	130
Conger, steamed	★ 92	4 oz.	92
Crab, without shells	★ 144	2 oz.	72
Crab paste	● 180	½ oz.	22
Dabs, fried	●● 224	4 oz.	224
Eels, stewed	●● 250	4 oz.	250
Eels, smoked	●● 380	4 oz.	380
Fish cake	●● 244	2 oz.	122
Flounder	★ 75	4 oz.	75
Gurnet	★ 104	4 oz.	104
Haddock, fried	●● 184	4 oz.	184
steamed	★ 84	4 oz.	84
Hake, steamed	★ 96	4 oz.	96
Halibut, steamed	● 112	4 oz.	112
Herring, fried	●● 268	4 oz.	268
Kippers	●● 190	4 oz.	190
Kippered, tinned	●● 270	2 oz.	135
Tinned in tomato sauce	●● 210	2 oz.	105
Kedgeree	●● 172	4 oz.	172
Lemon sole, steamed	★ 72	4 oz.	72
Lobster	★ 100	4 oz.	100
Lobster paste	● 180	½ oz.	22
Mackerel, fried	●● 156	4 oz.	156
Mullet, steamed	★ 96	4 oz.	96

	Calories in 4 oz.	Normal Helping	Calories in Normal Helping
Mussels, boiled without shells	★ 100	2 oz.	50
Oysters, raw without shells	★ 56	4 oz.	56
Pike	★ 90	4 oz.	90
Pilchards, tinned	●● 252	2 oz.	126
Plaice, steamed	★ 56	4 oz.	56
Prawns	★ 130	3 oz.	99
Prawn paste	● 180	½ oz.	22
Saithe, steamed	★ 96	4 oz.	96
Salmon, steamed	● 184	4 oz.	184
paste	● 200	½ oz.	25
tinned	● 156	4 oz.	156
Sardines, tinned	●● 336	2 oz.	168
paste	● 240	½ oz.	30
Shrimps	★ 128	2 oz.	64
paste	★ 200	½ oz.	25
Skate, fried	●● 228	4 oz.	228
Sole, steamed	★ 56	4 oz.	56
Sprats, smoked, grilled	●● 324	2 oz.	162
Trout, river, steamed	★ 110	4 oz.	110
Tuna Fish, tinned	● 228	3 oz.	171
Turbot, steamed	★ 76	4 oz.	76
Whiting	★ 68	4 oz.	68
Winkles, boiled, without shells	★ 108	4 oz.	108
Witch, steamed	★ 60	4 oz.	60

SOUPS

If you take the wrong soup you are in the soup!

Home-made soups

It is impossible to state the calorie value of home-made soups because of the various ingredients such as fat, flour, etc.

Tinned soups (not condensed)

	Calories in 4 oz.	Normal Helping	Calories in Normal Helping
Asparagus (creamed)	●● 68	5 oz.	85
Beef broth	● 48	5 oz.	60
Celery (creamed)	●● 72	5 oz.	90
Chicken (creamed)	●● 60	5 oz.	75
Chicken broth with rice	● 20	5 oz.	25
Kidney	●● 48	5 oz.	60
Mock Turtle	●● 56	5 oz.	60
Mulligatawny	●● 68	5 oz.	85
Mushroom (creamed)	●● 56	5 oz.	70
Onion (creamed)	●● 80	5 oz.	100
Oxtail	● 56	5 oz.	70
Green pea	●● 80	5 oz.	100
Scotch broth	●● 56	5 oz.	70
Tomato (creamed)	●● 80	5 oz.	100
Vegetable	● 52	5 oz.	65

SAUCES

" The English have a hundred religions but only one sauce. The French have a hundred sauces but only one religion."

(French proverb.)

For the slimmer, any religion, but no sauce!

	Calories in 4 oz.	Normal Helping	Calories in Normal Helping
Bread sauce	●● 128	2 oz.	64
Cheese sauce	●● 208	2 oz.	104
Cranberry sauce (sweet)	●● 208	2 oz.	104
Onion sauce	●● 100	2 oz.	50
Tomato Ketchup	●● 112	1 oz.	28
Tomato sauce	●● 84	2 oz.	42
White sauce	●● 164	2 oz.	82

MEAT, MEAT DISHES AND MEAT PRODUCTS

"Meat was made for mouth."
("Coriolanus"—W. Shakespeare.)

"Meat" for the slimmer, means meat only. The meat in meat pies, meat puddings, etc., often exists only in the name.

	Calories in 4 oz.	Normal Helping	Calories in Normal Helping
Beef:			
Beef dripping	●● 1048	½ oz.	131
Brain	★ 142	4 oz.	142
Brisket	★ 365	4 oz.	365
Corned beef (tinned)	★ 264	2 oz.	132
Frozen, raw	★ 172	6 oz.	258
Heart, raw	★ 150	6 oz.	225
Kidney, raw	★ 136	6 oz.	204
Liver, raw	★ 164	6 oz.	246
fried	● 320	4 oz.	320
paste	● 520	1 oz.	130
Silverside, boiled	★ 344	4 oz.	344
Sirloin, roast, fat	★ 436	4 oz.	436
roast, lean	★ 256	4 oz.	256
Steak, raw	★ 200	6 oz.	300
Sweetbread	★ 200	4 oz.	200
Tongue (tinned)	★ 340	2 oz.	170
Topside, roast	★ 364	4 oz.	364
Tripe, stewed	★ 116	4 oz.	116
Beef dishes:			
Steak pudding	●● 272	6 oz.	408
Beef stew	● 160	6 oz.	240
Hamburger	●● 412	2 oz.	206
Shepherd's pie	● 128	6 oz.	192
Sausage, fried	●● 324	2 oz.	162
Sausage roll	●● 536	2 oz.	268

		Calories in 4 oz.	Normal Helping	Calories in Normal Helping
Steak and kidney pie	●●	344	6 oz.	516
Toad in the hole	●●	328	4 oz.	328
Chicken:				
Raw meat	★	132	6 oz.	198
Raw liver	★	160	2 oz.	80
Boiled, with bone	★	152	4 oz.	152
Roast, with bone	★	116	4 oz.	116
Duck, roast with bone	●●	192	4 oz.	192
Goose:				
Liver	●●	264	4 oz.	264
Roast, with bone	●●	212	4 oz.	212
Hare, roast	★	148	4 oz.	148
Mutton:				
Chop, raw, with bone	●●	476	5 oz.	595
fried, with bone	●●	584	4 oz.	584
Leg, roast, with bone	●	382	4 oz.	382
Neck, raw	●	300	5 oz.	375
Shoulder, raw	●	300	5 oz.	375
Partridge, roast with bone	★	144	4 oz.	144
Pheasant, roast, with bone	★	152	4 oz.	152
Pigeon, roast, with bone	★	264	4 oz.	264
Pork:				
Bacon, raw, lean	●	360	2 oz.	180
Bacon, raw, fat	●●	520	2 oz.	260
Ham, boiled, lean	●	248	2 oz.	124
Ham, boiled, fat	●●	492	2 oz.	246
Luncheon meat	●●	328	2 oz.	164
Pork, lean	●	270	4 oz.	270
Pork, fat	●●	450	4 oz.	450
Sausage, fried	●●	372	2 oz.	186
Rabbit, stewed, with bone	★	104	4 oz.	104
Sausages, continental:				
Frankfurter	●	280	2 oz.	140

	Calories in 4 oz.	Normal Helping	Calories in Normal Helping
Salami	●● 520	2 oz.	260
Veal, roast	★ 264	4 oz.	264

VEGETABLES

An Austrian general in the 18th century said: "to win a war you need 1. MONEY; 2. MONEY; 3. MONEY." If he had been a dietician he would have told you that the safest way to slim is to eat 1. GREEN VEGETABLES; 2. GREEN VEGETABLES; 3. GREEN VEGETABLES.

	Calories in 4 oz.	Normal Helping	Calories in Normal Helping
Artichokes, boiled	★★ 16	4 oz.	16
Asparagus	★★ 20	4 oz.	20
Beans:			
baked, tinned	●● 112	4 oz.	112
broad, boiled	★ 48	4 oz.	48
butter, boiled	●● 104	4 oz.	104
haricot, boiled	●● 100	4 oz.	100
French beans	★★ 8	4 oz.	8
Beetroot, boiled	★ 52	4 oz.	52
Brussel sprouts, boiled	★★ 20	4 oz.	20
Cabbage	★★ 12	4 oz.	12
Carrots	★ 24	4 oz.	24
Cauliflower	★★ 28	4 oz.	28
Celery	★★ 12	4 oz.	12
Chicory	★★ 12	4 oz.	12
Cucumber	★★ 12	4 oz.	12
Leeks	★★ 36	4 oz.	36
Lentils, dried	●● 336	2 oz.	168
Lettuce	★★ 12	2 oz.	6
Marrow	★★ 10	4 oz.	10
Mushroom, raw	★★ 8	2 oz.	4
fried	●● 248	2 oz.	124

150 THE SLIMMING SECRET

	Calories in 4 oz.	Normal Helping	Calories in Normal Helping
✓ Onions, boiled	★★ 16	4 oz.	16
fried	●● 404	2 oz.	202
Parsley	★★ 24	¼ oz.	1–2
✓ Parsnips	● 56	4 oz.	56
Peas, fresh, raw	●● 72	4 oz.	72
dried	●● 312	2 oz.	156
tinned	●● 96	4 oz.	96
✓ Potatoes, boiled	● 92	4 oz.	92
mashed	●● 136	4 oz.	136
roast	●● 140	4 oz.	140
chips	●● 272	4 oz.	272
crisp	●● 636	2 oz.	318
Radishes	★★ 16	2 oz.	8
Spinach, boiled	★★ 28	4 oz.	28
✓ Swedes, boiled	★ 20	4 oz.	20
Sweet potatoes, boiled	● 92	4 oz.	92
✓ Tomatoes	★ 16	4 oz.	16
✓ Turnips	★ 20	4 oz.	20
Watercress	★★ 16	1 oz.	4

PUDDINGS

If you would cut out your pudding at lunch and dinner, and replace it with fresh fruit such as apples, oranges, etc., you have not only taken the first step but the first mile towards slimness.

	Calories in 4 oz.	Normal Helping	Calories in Normal Helping
Apple pudding	●●● 272	3 oz.	204
Apple pie	●●● 216	3 oz.	162
✓ Blancmange	●●● 136	4 oz.	136
Bread and butter pudding	●●● 184	3 oz.	138

THE SLIMMING SECRET

	Calories in 4 oz.	Normal Helping	Calories in Normal Helping
Custard, baked	●● 128	2 oz.	64
sauce	●● 136	2 oz.	68
Date pudding, tinned	●●● 340	3 oz.	255
Dumpling	●●● 236	3 oz.	177
Jam roll, baked	●●● 460	3 oz.	345
Jelly	●● 92	3 oz.	69
Pancakes	●●● 340	3 oz.	255
Plum pudding, tinned	●●● 360	3 oz.	270
Rice pudding	●●● 168	4 oz.	168
Semolina pudding	●●● 148	4 oz.	148
Tapioca pudding	●●● 148	4 oz.	148
Treacle pudding, tinned	●●● 364	3 oz.	273
Trifle	●●● 172	3 oz.	129
Yorkshire pudding	●● 252	2 oz.	126

FRUIT AND FRUIT PRODUCTS

"Half an orange tastes as sweet as a whole one."
(Chinese proverb.)

	Calories in 4 oz.	Normal Helping	Calories in Normal Helping
Almonds	●● 680	1 oz.	170
Almond paste	●● 560	1 oz.	140
Apples, raw	★ 60	4 oz.	60
Apples, dried	●● 268	2 oz.	134
Apple juice, tinned	● 60	8 oz.	120
Apple sauce, sweet	●● 80	2 oz.	40
Apricots, fresh	★ 32	4 oz.	32
Apricots, dried	●● 208	2 oz.	104
Apricots, tinned, sweet	●● 68	4 oz.	68
Apricot jam	●● 296	1 oz.	74
Avocado pears	●● 200	4 oz.	200
Bananas	●● 88	4 oz.	88
Blackberries, fresh	★ 30	4 oz.	30

	Calories in 4 oz.	Normal Helping	Calories in Normal Helping
Blackberries, tinned	● 80	4 oz.	80
Blackcurrants, raw	★ 24	4 oz.	24
Blackcurrant juice	● 50	8 oz.	100
Brazil nuts	●● 720	1 oz.	180
Cantaloupes	★ 20	4 oz.	20
Cashew nuts, roasted	●● 648	1 oz.	162
Cherries, fresh	★ 52	4 oz.	52
Cherries, tinned	●● 95	4 oz.	95
Cherries, candied	●● 270	1 oz.	68
Chestnuts, raw	●● 200	2 oz.	100
Chestnuts, roasted	●● 240	2 oz.	120
Cobnuts	●● 452	2 oz.	226
Coconuts, fresh	●● 416	2 oz.	208
Coconuts, desiccated	●● 720	1 oz.	180
Cranberries, fresh	★ 20	2 oz.	10
Cranberry sauce, sweet	●● 208	2 oz.	104
Currant jam	●● 296	1 oz.	74
Damsons, raw	★ 40	4 oz.	40
Damson jam	●● 296	1 oz.	74
Dates, dried, without stone	●● 280	2 oz.	140
Figs, fresh	★ 48	4 oz.	48
Figs, dried	●● 240	2 oz.	120
Gooseberries, fresh	★ 40	4 oz.	40
Gooseberries, tinned in syrup	●● 95	4 oz.	95
Grapes, black	● 56	4 oz.	56
Grapes, white	● 72	4 oz.	72
Grapefruit (without sugar)	★ 24	4 oz.	24
Grapefruit juice	● 45	8 oz.	90
Grapefruit, tinned in syrup	●● 70	4 oz.	70
Greengages	★ 52	4 oz.	52
Honeydew melon	★ 24	4 oz.	24

THE SLIMMING SECRET

	Calories in 4 oz.	Normal Helping	Calories in Normal Helping
Lemon	★ 16		
Loganberries, fresh	★ 20	4 oz.	20
Loganberries, tinned, sweet	●● 120	4 oz.	120
Nectarines	★ 32	4 oz.	32
Olives, without stones	● 120	1 oz.	30
Oranges	★ 32	5 oz.	40
Orange juice	● 70	8 oz.	140
Orange marmalade	●● 296	1 oz.	74
Peaches, fresh	★ 44	4 oz.	44
Peaches, dried	●● 244	2 oz.	122
Peaches, tinned	●● 80	4 oz.	80
Peanuts, roasted	●● 640	1 oz.	160
Peanut butter	●● 660	½ oz.	82
Pears, fresh	★ 44	4 oz.	44
Pears, dried	●● 180	2 oz.	90
Pears, tinned, sweet	●● 80	4 oz.	80
Pineapple, fresh	● 52	4 oz.	52
Pineapple, tinned, sweet	●● 72	4 oz.	72
Pineapple juice	● 75	8 oz.	150
Plums, fresh	★ 40	4 oz.	40
Plums, tinned, sweet	●● 80	4 oz.	80
Plum jam	●● 296	1 oz.	74
Pomegranates	● 100	5 oz.	125
Prunes, dried, raw	●● 150	2 oz.	75
Raisins, dried	●● 280	1 oz.	70
Raspberries, fresh	★ 28	4 oz.	28
Raspberries, tinned, sweet	●● 110	4 oz.	110
Raspberry juice	● 50	8 oz.	100
Raspberry jam	●● 296	1 oz.	74
Rhubarb, raw	★ 8	4 oz.	8
Strawberries, fresh	★ 28	4 oz.	28

154 THE SLIMMING SECRET

	Calories in 4 oz.	Normal Helping	Calories in Normal Helping
Strawberries, tinned, sweet	●● 125	4 oz.	125
Strawberry Juice	● 35	8 oz.	70
Strawberry jam	●● 296	1 oz.	74
Sultanas, dried	●● 284	1 oz.	71
Tangerines	★ 40	3 oz.	30
Walnuts (without shells)	●● 624	1 oz.	156
Watermelon	★ 35	4 oz.	35

SUGAR, SWEETS AND CHOCOLATES

Overweight is bitter, but the way to it is often sweet!

	Calories in 4 oz.	Normal Helping	Calories in Normal Helping
Boiled sweets	●●● 372	1 oz.	93
Chewing gum	●●	1 piece	7
Chocolate, milk	●●● 668	1 oz.	167
Chocolate, plain	●●● 620	1 oz.	155
Fondant	●●● 400	1 oz.	100
Fudge	●●● 440	1 oz.	110
Fruit gums	●● 196	1 oz.	49
Glucose, liquid	●●● 360	4 oz.	360
Honey	●●● 328	1 oz.	82
Ice cream	●●● 224	2 oz.	112
Jam	●● 296	1 oz.	74
Jelly (sweet)	●●● 292	2 oz.	146
Lemon curd	●●● 344	1 oz.	86
Marmalade	●● 296	1 oz.	74
Sugar	●●● 448	1 tsp.	30
Syrup	●●● 336	1 oz.	84
Toffees	●●● 460	1 oz.	115
Treacle	●●● 292	1 oz.	73

DRINKS

Watch the sugar and the milk because they can turn a harmless drink into a dangerous one!

BEVERAGES (NON-ALCOHOLIC)

	Calories in 4 oz.	Normal Helping	Calories in Normal Helping
Bournvita (Powder)	●● 420		
Bournvita (without Sugar)			
¼ oz. or 1 tsp. + water	●		26
¼ oz. or 1 tsp. + 6 oz. milk	●●		146
¼ oz. + 1 oz. milk + water	●		46
Bovril	★ 92	½ oz.	12
Cocoa (Powder)	●● 512		
Cocoa (without Sugar)			
¼ oz. or 1 tsp. + water	●		32
¼ oz. or 1 tsp. + 6 oz. milk	●●		152
¼ oz. + 1 oz. milk + water	●		52
Coffee	0		
Coffee (without Sugar)			
+ water	★		0
+ 6 oz. milk	●●		120
+ 1 oz. milk + water	★		20
Horlick (Powder)	●● 452		
Horlick (without Sugar)			
¼ oz. or 1 tsp. + water	●		28
¼ oz. or 1 tsp. + 6 oz. milk	●●		148
¼ oz. + 1 oz. milk + water	●		48
Lemon squash	●● 144		
Marmite	★★ 8	½ oz.	1

	Calories in 4 oz.	Normal Helping	Calories in Normal Helping
Milk	●● 80	8 oz.	160
Orange Squash	●● 160		
Ovaltine (Powder)	●● 436		
Ovaltine (without Sugar)			
¼ oz. or 1 tsp. + water	●		27
¼ oz. or 1 tsp. + 6 oz. milk	●●		147
¼ oz. + 1 oz. milk + water	●		47
Tea, Infusion	★ 0		
Tea (without Sugar)			
Tea + water	★ 0		0
Tea + 1 oz. milk	★		20

BEVERAGES (ALCOHOLIC)

No help to the slimmer. Reserve only for special occasions such as Christmas and anniversaries!

	Calories in 4 oz.	Normal Helping	Calories in Normal Helping
Ale	32 ●●	½ pint	80
Stout	40 ●●	½ pint	100
Burgundy	80 ●●	3 oz.	60
Cider (sweet)	48 ●●	½ pint	120
Hock	80 ●●	3 oz.	60
Port	180 ●●	3 oz.	135
Sherry	140 ●●	3 oz.	105
Vermouth	124 ●●	3 oz.	93
Brandy	280 ●●●	1 oz.	70
Gin	280 ●●●	1 oz.	70
Rum	280 ●●●	1 oz.	70
Whisky	280 ●●●	1 oz.	70

CONDIMENTS

	Calories in 4 oz.	Normal Helping	Calories in Normal Helping
Curry Powder	★		
Garlic	★		
Pepper	★	Calorie content negligible,	
Salt	★	safe for the slimmer.	
Vinegar	★		
Mustard	★		
Apple Chutney	●● 228	1 oz.	57
Tomato Chutney	●● 172	1 oz.	43
Tomato Ketchup	●● 112	1 oz.	28
Worcester Sauce	●● 96	1 oz.	24

Index

A
Advertisements, 77
Age, 20

B
Beverages, 155, 156
Biscuits, 140
Bread, 126, 137
Bread, Brown and White, 62
Bread, Protein, 64
Breakfast, 42
Butter, 65

C
Cakes, 140
Calories, 39 *et seq.*
Calorie Guide, 137 *et seq.*
Calorie Requirements, 51, 92 *et seq.*
Calorie Values, Learning, 52
Cereals, 139
Cheese, 49
Chocolates, 154
Climate, 20
Condiments, 157
Crispbreads, 64
Cyclamate, Sodium and Calcium, 60

D
Dairy Products, 141
Diabetes, 14, 18
Diet, High Fat, 46, 102
Diet, Vegetarian, 74
Diets, 1,000 calorie, 19
Diets, Crash, 95
Diets, Single Item, 100
Diuretics, 86
Drinks, 155
Drugs, 83 *et seq.*
Drugs, Appetite Suppressing, 84
Drugs, Hypoglycaemic, 87

E
Eggs, 47, 68, 69, 135
Exercise, 15, 20, 112

F
Fasting, 36, 37
Fat, 25, 29
Fats, 143
Fats, Saturated and Unsaturated, 108
Fish, 143
Frame, Large, Medium and Small, 32
Fruit, 151

G
Glands, 17 *et seq.*
Glucose, 66

H
Health Farms, 97
Heredity, 12 *et seq.*

INDEX

Honey, 67
Hormones, 86
Hunger, 36 *et seq.*

L

Laxatives, 86
Lemon, 68

M

Margarine, 65
Meat Foods, 45, 73, 147
Methylcellulose, 87
Middle Age Spread, 31
Milk, 70

P

Pastries, 140
Potatoes, 47
Preserved Foods, 71
Protein, 34
Puddings, 150

Q

Quacks, 89

S

Saccharine, 59
Sauces, 46
Salt, 27 *et seq.*
Slimming, difficulties, etc., 115 *et seq.*
Slimming foods, aids, 62 *et seq.*
Slimming methods, unsound and ineffective, 92 *et seq.*
Slimming Secret, The, 123 *et seq.*
Slimming, table, 31 *et seq.*
Snacks, 41, 129
Soups, 48, 145
Starvation. total, 99
Sugar. 14. 54 *et seq.*, 67, 154
Sugar Free Foods, 65
Sweets, 154

T

Thyroid. 17, 85
Toast, 64

V

Vegetables. 149
Vitamins, 80 *et seq.*

W

Water, 27 *et seq.*
Water, hot, 68
Weighing, 131
Weighing of foods, 50
Weight loss, calculating, 21 *et seq.*
Willpower, 51

Y

Yoghourt, 69

Uniform with this volume

The Right Way to Improve Your English
A gaily written explanation of the errors into which the beginner and experienced may so easily fall.
You can improve your English by studying this great work.

The Right Way to Conduct Meetings, Conferences and Discussions
The complete book for the Chairman, or for anyone involved in committee work or meetings of any kind. Contents include: The Chairman, The Secretary, Procedure, Votes of thanks, etc

Business Letters
During more than 30 years as a successful business man the author has perfected the art of writing business letters. He has also written thousands of other letters to Members of Parliament, organizations, newspapers, etc.

This is only a small selection from the wide range of *paperfronts*. A full catalogue can be had by sending S.A.E. to the address below.

ELLIOT RIGHT WAY BOOKS KINGSWOOD, SURREY, U.K.